Pg 20

UNDERSTANDING MALARIA AND LYME DISEASE

TROPICAL DISEASES - ETIOLOGY, PATHOGENESIS AND TREATMENTS

Additional books in this series can be found on Nova's website
under the Series tab.

Additional E-books in this series can be found on Nova's website
under the E-book tab.

PUBLIC HEALTH IN THE 21ST CENTURY

Additional books in this series can be found on Nova's website
under the Series tab.

Additional E-books in this series can be found on Nova's website
under the E-book tab.

TROPICAL DISEASES - ETIOLOGY, PATHOGENESIS
AND TREATMENTS

UNDERSTANDING MALARIA
AND LYME DISEASE

KRISTEN C. WALSCH
EDITOR

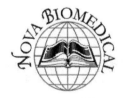

Nova Science Publishers, Inc.

New York

LIBRARY OF CONGRESS CATALOGING-IN-PUBLICATION DATA

Understanding malaria and lyme disease / editor, Kristen C. Walsch.
    p. ; cm.
  Includes index.
  ISBN 978-1-61761-435-4 (hardcover)
  1. Malaria. 2. Lyme disease. I. Walsch, Kristen C.
  [DNLM: 1. Malaria. 2. Lyme Disease. WC 750]
  RA644.M2U37 2010
  614.5'32--dc22
                                                                    2010029831

Published by Nova Science Publishers, Inc. † New York

CONTENTS

PREFACE

Malaria is a disease caused by a parasite that lives part of its life in humans and part in mosquitoes. Malaria remains one of the major killers of humans worldwide, threatening the lives of more than one-third of the world's population. It thrives in the tropical areas of Asia, Africa, and Central and South America, where it strikes millions of people. In the early 1970's, a mysterious clustering of arthritis cases occurred among children in Lyme, Connecticut, and surrounding towns. While scientists were busy describing signs and symptoms of Lyme disease to help doctors diagnose patients, they discovered that antibiotics were effective in its treatment and that the bite of the deer tick was the key to the spread of the disease. This book presents the most current research on the diagnosis, treatment and prevention of both malaria and Lyme disease

Chapter 1- Malaria is a disease caused by a **parasite*** that lives part of its life in humans and part in mosquitoes. Malaria remains one of the major killers of humans worldwide, threatening the lives of more than one- third of the world's population. It thrives in the tropical areas of Asia, Africa, and Central and South America, where it strikes millions of people. Each year 350 to 500 million cases of malaria occur worldwide. Sadly, more than 1 million of its victims, mostly young children, die yearly.

Although malaria has been virtually eradicated in the United States and other regions with temperate climates, it continues to affect hundreds of people in this country every year. The Centers for Disease Control and Prevention (CDC) estimates 1,200 cases of malaria are diagnosed each year in the United

---

* Note: Words in bold are defined in the glossary at the end of this booklet.

States. People who live in the United States typically get malaria during trips to malaria-**endemic** areas of the world.

Chapter 2- In 2008, malaria remained a serious problem in 109 countries, although it was eradicated almost 60 years ago in the United States. Malaria sickens an estimated 247 million people every year; of these, nearly 1 million die, mostly children younger than 5 years old. The disease is caused by a parasite that is transmitted to a person through the bite of a particular mosquito. Infection can lead to fever, muscle aches, and, without effective treatment, organ failure and sometimes death. Although approximately 40% of the world's population is at risk of malaria, most cases and deaths are in sub-Saharan Africa. In the past decade, the U.S. government and international community have increasingly recognized the impact of malaria prevention, treatment, and control on the health, economic development, and social well-being of people and communities in many developing countries.

Chapter 3- In the early 1970s, a mysterious clustering of arthritis cases occurred among children in Lyme, Connecticut, and surrounding towns. Puzzled medical experts eventually labeled the illness as a new disease, which they called Lyme disease. By the mid-1970s, scientists were busy describing signs and symptoms of Lyme disease to help doctors diagnose patients. Scientists eventually learned that antibiotics were an effective treatment, and that the bite of the deer tick was the key to the spread of disease.

None of these findings, however, happened overnight. In fact, it wasn't until 1981—through a bit of puzzle solving and keen recollection—that the cause of Lyme disease was identified and the connection between the deer tick and the disease was discovered.

In: Understanding Malaria and Lyme Disease   ISBN: 978-1-61761-435-4
Editors: Kristen C. Walsch   © 2010 Nova Science Publishers, Inc.

Chapter 1

UNDERSTANDING MALARIA: FIGHTING AN ANCIENT SCOURGE

U.S. Department of Health and Human Services

WHAT IS MALARIA?

Malaria is a disease caused by a **parasite**[*] that lives part of its life in humans and part in mosquitoes. Malaria remains one of the major killers of humans worldwide, threatening the lives of more than one-third of the world's population. It thrives in the tropical areas of Asia, Africa, and Central and South America, where it strikes millions of people. Each year 350 to 500 million cases of malaria occur worldwide. Sadly, more than 1 million of its victims, mostly young children, die yearly.

Although malaria has been virtually eradicated in the United States and other regions with temperate climates, it continues to affect hundreds of people in this country every year. The Centers for Disease Control and Prevention (CDC) estimates 1,200 cases of malaria are diagnosed each year in the United States. People who live in the United States typically get malaria during trips to malaria-**endemic** areas of the world.

---

[*] Note: Words in bold are defined in the glossary at the end of this booklet.

HISTORY OF MALARIA

Malaria has been around since ancient times. The early Egyptians wrote about it on papyrus, and the famous Greek physician Hippocrates described it in detail. It devastated invaders of the Roman Empire. In ancient Rome, as in other temperate climates, malaria lurked in marshes and swamps. People blamed the unhealthiness in these areas on rot and decay that wafted out on the foul air. Hence, the name is derived from the Italian, "*mal aria,*" or bad air. In 1880, the French scientist Alphonse Laveran discovered the real cause of malaria, the single-celled **Plasmodium** parasite. Almost 20 years later, scientists working in India and Italy discovered that **Anopheles** mosquitoes are responsible for transmitting malaria.

Historically, the United States is no stranger to the tragedy of malaria. This disease, then commonly known as "fever and ague," took a toll on early settlers. Historians believe that the incidence of malaria in this country peaked around 1875, but they estimate that by 1914 more than 600,000 new cases still occurred every year.

Malaria has been a significant factor in virtually all of the military campaigns involving the United States. In World War II and the Vietnam War, more personnel time was lost due to malaria than to bullets.

The discovery that malaria was transmitted by mosquitoes unleashed a flurry of ambitious public health measures designed to stamp out malaria. These measures were targeted at both the larval stages (which thrive in still waters, such as swamps) and adult stages of the insect. In some areas, such as the southern United States, draining swamps and changing the way land was used was somewhat successful in eliminating mosquitoes.

The pace of the battle accelerated rapidly when the insecticide DDT and the drug **chloroquine** were introduced during World War II. DDT was remarkably effective and could be sprayed on the walls of houses where adult *Anopheles* mosquitoes rested after feeding. Chloroquine has been a highly effective medicine for preventing and treating malaria.

In the mid-1950s, the World Health Organization (WHO) launched a massive worldwide campaign to eliminate malaria. At the beginning, the WHO program, which combined insecticide spraying and drug treatment, had many successes, some spectacular. In some areas, malaria was conquered completely, benefiting more than 600 million people, and was sharply curbed in the homelands of 300 million others.

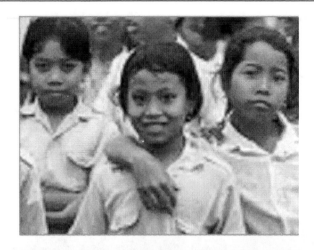

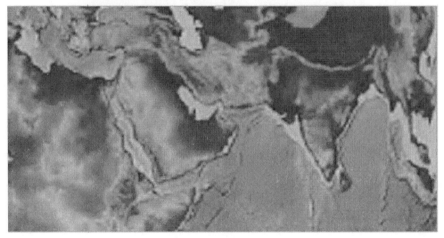

Difficulties soon developed, however. Some stumbling blocks were administrative, others financial. Even worse, nature intervened. More and more **strains** of *Anopheles* mosquitoes developed **resistance** to DDT and other insecticides, and the environmental impact of DDT was recognized. Meanwhile, the *Plasmodium* parasite became resistant to chloroquine, the mainstay of antimalarial drug treatment in humans.

Researchers estimate that infection rates increased by 40 percent between 1970 and 1997 in sub-Saharan Africa. To cope with this dangerous resurgence, public health workers carefully select prevention methods best suited to a particular environment or area. In addition to medicines and insecticides, they are making efforts to control mosquitoes, by draining swampy areas and filling them with dirt, as well as using window screens, mosquito netting, and insect repellents.

At the same time, scientists are intensively researching ways to develop better weapons against malaria, including

- Sophisticated techniques for tracking disease transmission worldwide
- More effective ways of treating malaria
- New ways, some quite ingenious, to control transmission of malaria by mosquitoes
- A vaccine for blocking malaria's development and spread

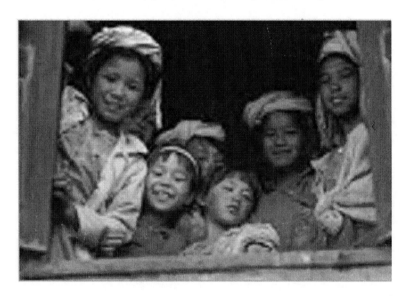

CAUSE OF MALARIA

Malaria is caused by a single-celled parasite from the **genus** *Plasmodium*. More than 100 different **species** of *Plasmodium* exist. They produce malaria in many types of animals and birds, as well as in humans.

Four species of *Plasmodium* commonly infect humans. Each one has a distinctive appearance under the microscope, and each one produces a somewhat different pattern of symptoms. Two or more species can live in the same area and infect a single person at the same time.

Plasmodium falciparum is responsible for most malaria deaths, especially in Africa. The infection can develop suddenly and produce several life-threatening complications. With prompt, effective treatment, however, it is almost always curable.

Plasmodium vivax, the most geographically widespread of the species, produces less severe symptoms. **Relapses,** however, can occur for up to 3 years, and chronic disease is debilitating. Once common in temperate climates, *P. vivax* is now found mostly in the tropics, especially throughout Asia.

Plasmodium malariae infections not only produce typical malaria symptoms but also can persist in the blood for very long periods, possibly decades, without ever producing symptoms. A person with asymptomatic (no symptoms) *P. malariae*, however, can infect others, either through blood donation or mosquito bites. *P. malariae* has been wiped out from temperate climates, but it persists in Africa.

Plasmodium ovale is rare, can cause relapses, and generally occurs in West Africa.

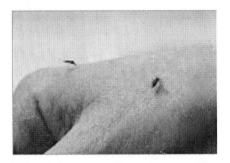

LIFE CYCLE OF THE MALARIA PARASITE

The human malaria parasite has a complex life cycle that requires both a human host and an insect host. In *Anopheles* mosquitoes, *Plasmodium* reproduces sexually (by merging the parasite's sex cells). In people, the parasite reproduces asexually (by cell division), first in liver cells and then, repeatedly, in red blood cells (RBCs).

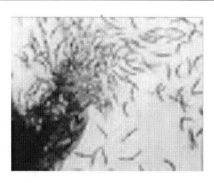

When an infected female *Anopheles* mosquito bites a human, it takes in blood. At the same time, it injects saliva that contains the infectious form of the parasite, the **sporozoite**, into a person's bloodstream [1].

[Numbers in brackets refer to Parasite Life Cycle diagram on pages 10–11.]

The thread-like sporozoite then invades a liver cell [2]. There, during the next week or two (depending on the *Plasmodium* species), each sporozoite develops into a **schizont**, a structure that contains thousands of tiny rounded **merozoites** (another stage of the parasite). When the schizont matures, it ruptures and releases the merozoites into the bloodstream [3].

Alternatively, some *P. vivax* and *P. ovale* sporozoites turn into **hypnozoites**, a form that can remain dormant in the liver for months or years. If they become active again, the hypnozoites develop into schizonts that then cause relapses in infected people.

Merozoites released from the liver upon rupture of schizonts rapidly invade RBCs, where they grow by consuming **hemoglobin** [4]. Within the RBC, most merozoites go through another round of asexual reproduction, again forming schizonts filled with yet more merozoites. When the schizont matures, the cell ruptures and merozoites burst out. The newly released merozoites invade other RBCs, and the infection continues its cycle until it is brought under control, either by medicine or the body's **immune system** defenses.

The *Plasmodium* parasite completes its life cycle through the mosquito when some of the merozoites that penetrate RBCs do not develop asexually into schizonts, but instead change into male and female sexual forms known as **gametocytes** [4]. These circulate in the person's bloodstream, awaiting the arrival of a blood- seeking female *Anopheles* mosquito [5].

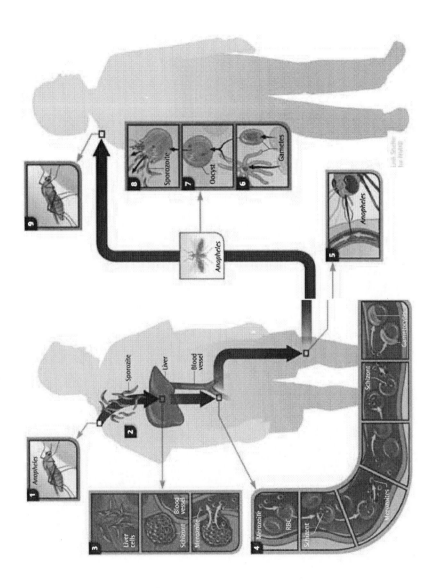

1 Anopheles

2 Sporozoite
Liver
Blood vessel

3 Liver cells
Blood vessel
Schizont
Merozoite

4 Merozoite
RBC
Schizont
Microgametes
Schizont
Gametocytes

5 Anopheles

Anopheles

6 Gametes

7 Oocyst

8 Sporozoite

9

When a female mosquito bites an infected person, it sucks up gametocytes along with blood. Once in the mosquito's stomach, the gametocytes develop into sperm-like male **gametes** or large, egg-like female gametes [6]. Fertilization produces an **oocyst** filled with infectious sporozoites [7]. When the oocyst matures, it ruptures and the thread-like sporozoites migrate, by the thousands, to the mosquito's salivary (saliva-producing) glands [8]. The cycle starts over again when the mosquito bites its next victim [9]

TRANSMISSION OF MALARIA

The malaria parasite typically is transmitted to people by mosquitoes belonging to the genus *Anopheles*. In rare cases, a person may contract malaria through contaminated blood, or a fetus may become infected by its mother during pregnancy.

Because the malaria parasite is found in RBCs, malaria can also be transmitted through blood transfusion, organ transplant, or the shared use of needles or syringes contaminated with blood. Malaria also may be transmitted from a mother to her fetus before or during delivery ("congenital" malaria).

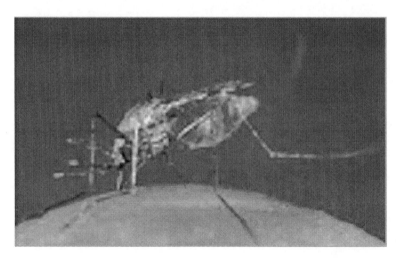

SPREAD OF MALARIA

Many biological and environmental factors shape the character of malaria in a given location. Nearly all the people who live in endemic areas are exposed to infection repeatedly. Those who survive malaria in childhood gradually build up some **immunity**. They may carry the infection, serving as reservoirs for transmission by mosquitoes without developing severe disease. In other areas, where the infection rate is low, people do not develop immunity because they rarely are exposed to the disease. This makes them more susceptible to the ravages of an **epidemic**. An epidemic can occur when conditions, such as those discussed below, allow the mosquito population to increase suddenly.

Effects of Climate

Climate affects both parasites and mosquitoes. Mosquitoes cannot survive in low humidity. Rainfall expands breeding grounds, and in many tropical areas, malaria cases increase during the rainy season. Mosquitoes must live long enough for the parasite to complete its development within them. Therefore, environmental factors that affect mosquito survival can influence malaria incidence.

Plasmodium parasites are affected by temperature—their development slows as the temperature drops. *P. vivax* stops developing altogether when the temperature falls below 60 degrees Fahrenheit. *P. falciparum* stops at somewhat higher temperatures. This effect explains why parasites can be found in temperate areas.

Effect of Human Intervention

People have worked for centuries to control malaria and were successful in eradicating it from most of North America early in the 20th century. Certain human activities, however, have inadvertently worsened the spread of malaria.

City conditions, for example, can create new places for mosquito **larvae** to develop. Agricultural practices also can affect mosquito breeding areas. Although the draining and drying of swamps gets rid of larval breeding sites, water-filled irrigation ditches may give mosquitoes another area to breed. In addition, because farmers use the same pesticides on their crops as those used against malaria **vector** mosquitoes, the problem of insecticide-resistant mosquitoes is growing. Modern transportation also contributes to the spread of the disease, moving travelers and occasionally mosquitoes between malaria-endemic and non-endemic regions.

Blood

Malaria is transmitted occasionally through transfusions of blood from infected individuals or sharing of needles to inject intravenous drugs, and can be transmitted from an infected pregnant woman to her unborn child. In the United States, however, transmission rarely occurs through blood transfusions, because blood donors are not allowed to donate for specified periods of time after traveling to or living in a malarious area.

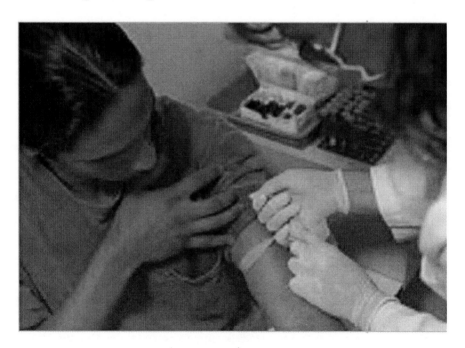

SYMPTOMS OF MALARIA

Malaria typically produces a string of recurrent attacks, or **paroxysms**, each of which has three stages— chills, followed by fever, and then sweating. Along with chills, the person is likely to have headache, malaise, fatigue, and muscular pains, and occasionally nausea, vomiting, and diarrhea. Within an hour or two, the body temperature rises, and the skin feels hot and dry. Then, as the body temperature falls, a drenching sweat begins. The person, feeling tired and weak, is likely to fall asleep.

The symptoms first appear some 10 to 16 days after the infectious mosquito bite and coincide with the bursting of infected RBCs. When many RBCs are infected and break at the same time, malaria attacks can recur at regular time periods— every 2 days for *P. vivax* malaria and *P. ovale*, and every 3 days for *P. malariae*.

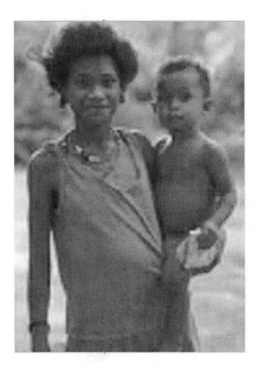

With *P. vivax* malaria, the person may feel fine between attacks. Even without treatment, the paroxysms subside in a few weeks. A person with *P. falciparum* malaria, however, is likely to feel miserable even between attacks and, without treatment, may die. One reason *P. falciparum* malaria is so

virulent is that the parasite can infect RBCs in all stages of development, leading to very high parasite levels in the blood. In contrast, *P. vivax* parasites infect only young RBCs, which means the number of parasites in the blood does not reach the same high levels as seen in *P. falciparum* infection.

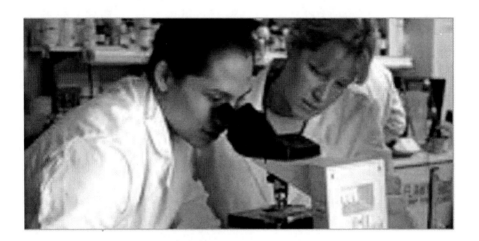

DIAGNOSING MALARIA

Health care providers should suspect malaria in anyone who has been in the tropics recently or received a blood transfusion, and who develops a fever and other signs that resemble the flu. They examine blood smears taken from a finger prick under a microscope to confirm the diagnosis. A "thick" smear makes it possible to examine a large amount of blood. Then, the species of parasite can be identified by looking at a corresponding "thin" smear. Because mixed infections are possible, these techniques are important for deciding the best treatment. For example, a person can be infected with *P. vivax* as well as the more dangerous *P. falciparum*. In the unusual event that parasites cannot be seen immediately in a blood smear, but the person's condition and prior activities strongly suggest malaria, a health care provider may decide to start treatment before being sure the person has malaria.

TREATING AND PREVENTING MALARIA

In most cases, health care providers can successfully treat people with malaria. To decide which medicine to use, they should try to identify the species of parasite responsible and the geographical location where the person was infected. Up-to-date information on the geography of malaria is available from international travel clinics, CDC, and WHO, including

Which species are present in which areas
Whether chloroquine-resistant parasites are present
Which seasons of the year carry the greatest risk

Before leaving home, anyone traveling to an area with malaria should consult a knowledgeable health care provider, an international travel clinic, a local health department, CDC, or WHO to obtain advice on what medicines to take before, during, and after the trip. Health risks for malaria vary with the destination, conditions of travel, and types of activities the traveler will undertake. A traveler who spends even a single night in a malaria-endemic area risks getting infected.

CDC and WHO have information on how to limit contact with mosquitoes, as well as current guidelines on antimalarial drugs.

RESEARCH ON MALARIA

As the lessons of the past decades have convincingly demonstrated, conquering malaria is difficult. No one anticipates a quick victory even if new malaria drugs hit the market, or a vaccine proves highly successful. Rather, researchers and health planners expect their best chances lie in a many-sided attack, drawing upon a variety of weapons suited to local environments. Skillfully combining several approaches, both old and new, may at last make it possible to outmaneuver these persistent and deadly parasites.

Medicines

Medicines to treat malaria have been around for thousands of years. Perhaps the best known of the traditional remedies is **quinine**, which is derived from the bark of the cinchona tree. The Spanish learned about quinine from Peruvian Indians in the 1600s. Export of quinine to Europe, and later the United States, was a lucrative business until World War II cut off access to the world supply of cinchona bark. In the 1940s, an intensive research program to find alternatives to quinine gave rise to the manufacture of chloroquine and numerous other chemical compounds that became the forerunners of modern antimalarial drugs.

Chloroquine was the third most widely used drug in the world until the mid-1990s. It is cheap to manufacture, easy to give, and does not cause problems for most people. Unfortunately, chloroquine-resistant malaria parasites have developed and have spread to most areas of the world. From the 1950s to the present, chloroquine resistance gradually spread to nearly all *P. falciparum* malaria-endemic regions.

In the 1960s, the U.S. Government, WHO, and other agencies launched a massive search for new antimalarial drugs. In addition, many doctors treating people in Asia are using yet another new family of drugs based on the parent drug artemisinin, an extract of the Chinese herbal remedy qinghaosu.

Unfortunately, malaria parasites in many geographic regions have become resistant to alternative drugs, many of which were discovered only in the last 30 years. Even quinine, the long-lived mainstay of malaria treatment, is losing its effectiveness in certain areas.

To address the problem of drug-resistant malaria, scientists are conducting research on the genetic mechanisms that enable *Plasmodium* parasites to avoid the toxic effects of malaria drugs. Understanding how those mechanisms work should enable scientists to develop new medicines or alter existing ones to make drug resistance more difficult. By knowing how the parasite survives and interacts with the human host during each distinct phase of its development, researchers also hope to develop drugs that attack the parasite at different stages.

For example, National Institute of Allergy and Infectious Diseases (NIAID) scientists are studying the **molecules** on host cells that malaria parasites use to attach to and enter the cells. Malaria parasites invade various tissues such as skin, blood, liver, gut, and salivary glands of human and mosquito hosts, which means the parasites must be able to attach to a diverse array of molecules (called receptors) on the outside of host cells. By determining the three-dimensional structures of these receptors, scientists hope to determine exactly how the parasites target particular types of cells, which may reveal new targets for antimalarial drugs.

NIAID scientists are also working to understand how *P. falciparum* has adapted to survive and grow within RBCs. An important category of these adaptations involves the trafficking of nutrients across various membranes of the infected RBC. To this end, researchers have identified two nutrient channels unique to the infected cell and plan to study these further to identify their genetic bases and to develop detailed mechanistic models of nutrient transport. With these models, they may be able to design channel blockers that interfere with the parasite's ability to acquire needed nutrients. These blockers may prove to be novel and useful drugs for treating malaria.

Finally, NIAID scientists are unraveling the mechanisms of natural resistance to malaria infection, which is yielding valuable information for new antimalarial drug development. For example, in regions of West Africa, up to one-fourth of children carry hemoglobin C, a variant of hemoglobin that can reduce the risk of severe and fatal malaria by as much as 80 percent. The way hemoglobin C protects people, however, had been puzzling.

NIAID scientists and their team of international collaborators discovered that hemoglobin C protects against malaria by affecting a key parasite protein, called PfEMP 1, that malaria parasites normally place on host RBCs in knoblike protrusions. The protruding proteins then make the infected RBCs stick to the lining of blood vessels in the brain and other critical tissues, which causes inflammation and circulatory obstruction. Hemoglobin C alters the membrane of RBCs so that the parasites cannot place PfEMP 1 normally at the cell surface. Thus, these RBCs are less able to adhere to vessel walls, which reduces disease severity. Other hemoglobin variants, such as the sickle-cell mutation, may protect against malaria by a similar mechanism. These findings suggest that interventions affecting the display of PfEMP 1 may reduce the impact of malaria.

Mosquito Control

The appearance and spread of insecticide-resistant mosquitoes, as well as stricter environmental regulations, now limit the effectiveness and use of the insecticide DDT, the mainstay of 1950s and 1960s malaria eradication programs.

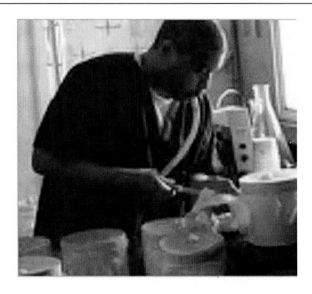

More recently, researchers have found that mosquito netting soaked with pyrethroid insecticides, which prevent mosquitoes from making contact with humans, significantly reduces malaria transmission. Therefore, as part of its Roll Back Malaria program, WHO is promoting widespread use of insecticide-treated mosquito netting in malaria-endemic areas. Still, in some parts of Western Africa, mosquitoes have become resistant to pyrethroid insecticide used to treat the nets. Although scientists do not think this development is a serious limitation yet, it points out the need to continue research to identify new tools for mosquito control.

Vaccines

Research studies conducted in the 1960s and 1970s showed that experimental vaccination of people with **attenuated** malaria parasites can effectively immunize them against getting another malaria infection. Current methods to develop vaccines based on weakened or killed malaria parasites are technically difficult and do not readily lend themselves to being produced commercially. Therefore, much of the research on vaccines has focused on identifying specific components or **antigens** of the malaria parasite that can stimulate protective immunity.

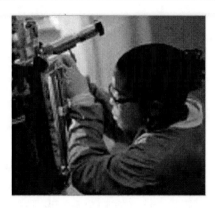

In 1997, NIAID launched a Plan for Research to Accelerate Development of Malaria Vaccines based on four cornerstones.

- Establishing a resource center to provide scientists worldwide with well-characterized reference and research reagents
- Increasing support for discovery of new vaccine candidates
- Increasing capacity to produce vaccine candidates at the quality and quantity that will be required for clinical trials
- Establishing research and training centers in endemic areas where potential vaccines may undergo clinical trials.

The NIAID Malaria Vaccine Development Branch (MVDB) is part of the institute's initiative to respond to the global need for malaria vaccines. MVDB has developed and produced several proteins on parasite antigens sequences to include in candidate malaria vaccines. This work involves collaborations with colleagues from other Federal agencies, the private sector, and academia in the United States and throughout the world, as well as assistance from a variety of partners, such as the U.S. Agency for International Development and the Malaria Vaccine Initiative.

Researchers are evaluating six potential vaccine antigens in human Phase I vaccine trials, either alone or in combinations, using three adjuvants, or vaccine boosters. The trials are under way both in the United States and in an endemic population in Mali in collaboration with the University of Bamako, Mali. These vaccine trials form part of a clinical development plan working towards Phase II trials in an endemic area that will determine if these vaccines are able to make a substantial impact on parasite growth or transmission.

Under these and other programs, scientists are conducting research to understand the nature of protective immunity in humans and methods to induce protective immune responses with malaria antigens.

Genome Sequencing

Genome sequencing, the process that allows scientists to determine an **organism's** genetic blueprint, is accelerating the discovery of new targets for drugs, vaccines, and diagnostic tests for malaria and other infectious diseases. By examining those blueprints, researchers can determine the genes that control a broad range of an organism's biological properties, such as feeding, reproducing, and adapting to its environment.

The complete genome sequences for the *Anopheles gambiae* mosquito and the *P. falciparum* parasite were published in 2002. Researchers are currently sequencing the genomes of other *Plasmodium* species. These advances mark a milestone in malaria research. Combined with the completed human genome sequence, scientists have the complete genetic blueprints for the malaria parasite and both of its hosts. Researchers are now using that information to learn more about how *Plasmodium* survives within people and mosquitoes, and to discover new ways to diagnose, prevent, and treat the disease.

Other Research Efforts

As with other diseases of worldwide importance, a critical aspect of our future ability to control malaria will depend on the skills and expertise of scientists, health care providers, and public health specialists working in malaria-endemic regions. Therefore, strengthening the research capabilities of scientists in these areas is another major focus of these efforts.

Through its support of the Malaria Research and Reference Reagent Resource Center (MR4), NIAID provides well-characterized research materials to scientists in malaria-endemic areas. NIAID also works closely with national and international organizations involved in malaria research and control. In addition, NIAID was a founding member of the Multilateral Initiative on Malaria, which emphasizes strengthening research capacity in Africa.

GLOSSARY

Anopheles—the genus of mosquito that transmits malaria. This genus includes many species that are vectors for malaria transmission.

antigen—a molecule on a microbe that identifies it as foreign to the immune system and stimulates the immune system to attack it.

attenuated—treated in such a way as to decrease the ability of the parasite to cause infection or disease.

chloroquine—the primary drug used to treat malaria since 1945. It is no longer effective against a growing number of strains of *P. falciparum* malaria.

endemic—area where malaria is constantly present.

epidemic—a disease outbreak that affects many people in a region at the same time.

gametes—reproductive elements, male and female.

gametocytes—precursors of the sexual forms of the malaria parasite, which release either male or female gametes within the stomach of the mosquito.

genus—a category of organisms.

hemoglobin—the oxygen-carrying part of red blood cells.

hypnozoite—a form of the malaria parasite that remains inactive within the liver and can produce relapses of malaria.

immune system—a complex network of specialized cells, tissues, and organs that defends the body against attacks by disease-causing microbes.

immunity—the protection generated by the body's immune system in response to invasion by "foreign" invaders, including bacteria, parasites, and viruses.

larvae—immature wingless forms of insects such as mosquitoes.

merozoite—the form of the malaria parasite that invades human red blood cells.

molecules—building blocks of a cell. Some examples are proteins, fats, and carbohydrates.

oocyst—a parasite stage within the mosquito, produced by the union of male and female gametes.

organism—an individual living thing.

parasite—plants or animals that live, grow, and feed on or within another living organism.

paroxysm—an attack of a disease that is likely to recur at periodic intervals.

Plasmodium—the genus of the parasite that causes malaria.

quinine—a drug, originally extracted from tree bark, which was the only available antimalarial treatment for nearly 300 years.

relapses—recurrences of a disease some time after it apparently has been controlled or cured.

resistance—the ability of an organism to develop strains that are impervious to specific threats to their existence.

schizont—a developmental form of the parasite that contains many merozoites.

species—organisms in the same genus that have similar characteristics.

sporozoite—the infectious form of the parasite, which is injected into people by a feeding mosquito.

strain—a genetic variant within a species.

vector—the organism, typically an insect, that transmits an infectious agent to its alternate host, typically a vertebrate. In human malaria, the vectors of the parasite are mosquitoes; the "carriers" or "hosts" are humans.

virulent—toxic, causing disease.

In: Understanding Malaria and Lyme Disease   ISBN: 978-1-61761-435-4
Editors: Kristen C. Walsch   © 2010 Nova Science Publishers, Inc.

Chapter 2

THE PRESIDENT'S MALARIA INITIATIVE AND OTHER U.S. GLOBAL EFFORTS TO COMBAT MALARIA: BACKGROUND, ISSUES FOR CONGRESS, AND RESOURCES

Kellie Moss

SUMMARY

In 2008, malaria remained a serious problem in 109 countries, although it was eradicated almost 60 years ago in the United States. Malaria sickens an estimated 247 million people every year; of these, nearly 1 million die, mostly children younger than 5 years old. The disease is caused by a parasite that is transmitted to a person through the bite of a particular mosquito. Infection can lead to fever, muscle aches, and, without effective treatment, organ failure and sometimes death. Although approximately 40% of the world's population is at risk of malaria, most cases and deaths are in sub-Saharan Africa. In the past decade, the U.S. government and international community have increasingly recognized the impact of malaria prevention, treatment, and control on the health, economic development, and social well-being of people and communities in many developing countries.

U.S. policymakers have demonstrated a strong interest in combating malaria. In May 2003, Congress passed the United States Leadership Against

HIV/AIDS, Tuberculosis, and Malaria Act (P.L. 108-25), which states, among other things, that a major objective of the U.S. foreign assistance program is to provide aid for the prevention, control, and cure of malaria, and authorizes funds to carry out these programs. In 2004-2006, congressional hearings on U.S. global efforts to combat malaria, especially those of the United States Agency for International Development (USAID), discussed USAID policies associated with purchasing and distributing commodities like antimalarial drugs and insecticides, providing technical assistance, and promoting program transparency, and questioned the U.S. strategy for fighting global malaria. In July 2008, Congress passed the Tom Lantos and Henry J. Hyde United States Global Leadership Against HIV/AIDS, Tuberculosis, and Malaria Reauthorization Act (P.L. 110-293), which authorizes $5 billion from FY2009 through FY2013 for U.S. global malaria efforts. It also directs the President to develop a comprehensive, five-year U.S. government strategy to fight global malaria, and authorizes the position of the U.S. Global Malaria Coordinator to oversee and coordinate all U.S. government programs to fight malaria globally.

In June 2005, President George W. Bush announced the President's Malaria Initiative (PMI), a $1.2 billion, five-year initiative to reduce the number of malaria-related deaths in 15 sub-Saharan African countries by 50% by 2010. U.S. global malaria efforts include PMI, which is led by USAID and implemented in conjunction with the Centers for Disease Control and Prevention (CDC); other USAID malaria programs; and CDC's global malaria activities.

From FY2004 through FY2008, USAID and CDC received $915 million for U.S. global malaria programs, of which more than $484 million was directed to PMI. During this time, the U.S. government also contributed more than $3 billion to the Global Fund to Fight AIDS, Tuberculosis, and Malaria (Global Fund), which funds malaria projects among other projects. For FY2009, Congress has appropriated $391.9 million for U.S. global malaria programs and $900 million for U.S. contributions to the Global Fund.

This report provides background on malaria's cause, consequences, and impact as well as ways to prevent, treat, and control it. The report discusses not only USAID malaria programs and CDC's Malaria Branch, but also efforts to coordinate these bilateral efforts with multilateral efforts. The report describes funding for U.S. efforts to fight malaria. Finally, it raises possible issues related to these efforts for the 111th Congress, such as U.S. malaria funding levels, U.S. program priorities and strategies, access to commodities, and oversight of U.S. programs.

INTRODUCTION

Malaria's impact is widespread. Although eradicated almost 60 years ago in the United States, malaria remained a serious problem in 109 countries in 2008. Malaria is a disease caused by a parasite that is transmitted to a person through the bite of a particular mosquito. It can lead to fever, muscle aches, and, without effective treatment, sometimes death. Globally, an estimated 247 million people become ill due to malaria every year; of these, nearly 1 million die, mostly children younger than five years old. Approximately 40% of the world's population is at risk of malaria, but most cases and deaths are in sub-Saharan Africa.[1]

In the past decade, the U.S. government and international community have increasingly recognized malaria prevention, treatment, and control as a fundamental factor in community health and economic growth in developing countries. Despite global efforts to eradicate malaria in many regions in the 1950s and 1960s, the 1990s saw a resurgence of the disease after national and international investments in malaria research and control declined. Many leaders expressed their growing concern about the negative impact of high rates of malaria infection and death on many developing countries during high-level meetings and summits, including the United Nations (U.N.) General Assembly. Many U.S. policymakers have, likewise, demonstrated a strong interest in combating malaria. In recent years, Congress has passed legislation that states that a major objective of the U.S. foreign assistance program is to provide aid for the prevention, control, and cure of malaria; required the development of a U.S. global malaria strategy; and appropriated increased funding for U.S. programs that fight the disease globally. At the same time, the U.S. government reorganized many U.S. malaria programs and changed program policies to emphasize funding for commodities (such as antimalarial drugs and mosquito nets), their effective distribution and implementation, and monitoring and evaluation activities.

This report provides background on malaria's cause, consequences, and impact as well as key interventions for its prevention, control, and treatment. It examines congressional activities related to global malaria, and then it describes U.S. programs through the U.S. Agency for International Development (USAID) and the Centers for Disease Control and Prevention (CDC) that address the disease internationally. The report describes U.S. funding for these activities. It also raises possible issues for Congress related to U.S. funding levels, U.S. program priorities and strategies, access to and effectiveness of commodities, and oversight of U.S. programs. Except for

CDC operational and applied research, this report does not describe U.S. government activities related to malaria research.[2] Appendix A provides a glossary of acronyms and abbreviations used in the body of this report. Appendix B lists additional key books, articles, and reports on malaria.

MALARIA BACKGROUND

Malaria is a complex disease that has been successfully eradicated in some parts of the world, including the United States. However, in other areas, eradication efforts have failed or not been attempted at all. Experts agree that it is important to understand not only the disease and its impact but also the recent history of international malaria efforts if ongoing efforts are going to succeed in controlling malaria where past programs did not.

Cause, Consequences, and Impact of Malaria[3]

Malaria is caused by *Plasmodium* parasites, which are transmitted to humans through the bite of infected female *Anopheles* mosquitoes.[4] First, these parasites multiply in the liver; then they infect red blood cells. A week or two after someone is bitten by an infected mosquito, initial symptoms appear, including fever, shivering, headache, nausea, vomiting, muscle aches and fatigue. Without effective treatment, these symptoms may rapidly progress to include organ failure, delirium, convulsions, coma, and sometimes death.

Malaria infects people of all ages, but some groups — pregnant women, infants and young children, and people living with HIV/AIDS — are more vulnerable to the disease. Most cases and deaths, including more than 9 out of 10 child deaths from malaria, are in sub-Saharan Africa, but other regions of the world, including parts of Asia, Latin America, the Middle East and Europe, are also affected (see Figure 1). Those countries that have a fairly constant number of cases throughout the year are considered malaria endemic countries. In 2008, 109 countries were considered malaria endemic; of these, 45 were in sub-Saharan Africa.

The incidence of malaria appears to correlate to many other factors affecting the health, economic development, and social well being of people and communities in many developing countries. High rates of malaria in a developing country may negatively affect economic growth and demand a great proportion of public health resources. In 2003, 25-40% of all outpatient clinic visits and 20-50% of hospital admissions in malaria endemic countries in Africa were for malaria. With the scale-up of malaria programs in many malaria endemic countries, some countries report fewer malaria-related hospital admissions. Often, poor or marginalized populations are disproportionately affected by malaria. While experts debate whether poverty leads to malaria or malaria leads to poverty, some suggest that high rates of malaria can continue the cycle of poverty by draining financial resources and contributing to absenteeism from schools or the workplace. Additionally, many malaria deaths in Africa occur among populations affected by conflicts, which may experience malaria outbreaks due to disruptions in healthcare and malaria control efforts as well as exposure to different malaria transmission patterns.

Prevention, Treatment, and Control of Malaria

Experts agree that preventing malaria infections as well as accurately diagnosing and treating malaria quickly are essential to control the spread of malaria. Four key strategies for combating malaria are:[5]

- **Effective** Treatment **with ACTs**: Treating malaria early and with effective drugs shortens its duration and prevents complications and most malaria-related deaths. Several drugs are used to treat malaria, and they vary in cost, availability, and effectiveness. In most areas, donors or Ministries of Health prefer to use artemisinin-based combination therapies (ACTs), which succeed generations of antimalarial drugs, including chloroquine, that have become less effective in fighting the malaria parasite due to increased drug resistance. ACTs are made up of an artemisinin drug and one or more additional antimalarial drugs; using antimalarial drugs in combination rather than singly reduces the likelihood that the malaria parasite will develop resistance to a drug.
- **IPTp**: In many malaria-endemic areas, women may be given intermittent preventive treatment of malaria during pregnancy (IPTp) — spaced doses of the drug sulfadoxine-pyrimethamine (SP) — in order to reduce the rates of malaria- related low birth weights in newborn babies and malaria-related anemia in pregnant women.6
- **IRS**: Another way of reducing the transmission of malaria is through indoor residual spraying (IRS) — spraying the inside walls of houses

with a long-acting insecticide. By controlling the presence of malaria-infected mosquitoes through IRS, malaria transmission can be reduced or interrupted. Several types of insecticides are used in the environment to control mosquitoes, and, like antimalarial drugs, they vary in cost, availability, and effectiveness.

- ITNs: The use of insecticide-treated mosquito nets (ITNs) is another strategy to prevent malaria-infected mosquitoes from biting people and transmitting the disease. These nets protect individuals or families from malaria when people sleep under nets hung over their beds. The nets also kill the mosquitoes. These nets usually retain their insecticidal properties for up to six months, depending on how frequently they are washed, without re-treatment. Some long-lasting insecticidal nets (LLINs) have insecticide incorporated into their fibers and last for up to 3 years.

However, the appropriate mix of prevention and treatment interventions may vary according to local conditions, including the presence of parasite resistance to antimalarial drugs (including ACTs and SP) and mosquito resistance to insecticides. USAID's selected interventions in a country also vary based on the pattern of disease transmission, the age and pregnancy status of infected persons, and whether activities are feasible and sustainable.[7]

Recent International Attention on Malaria

Malaria prevention, treatment, and control, which is increasingly recognized as a fundamental component of community health and economic growth in developing countries, has re-emerged as a major international concern in the past decade. In the 1950s and 1960s, multilateral efforts to eradicate malaria globally and in specific countries increased; some programs experienced setbacks or failure while others had more success. However, sub-Saharan Africa was largely excluded from these efforts. Reasons given for this vary: the region's high malaria infection rates; the costs associated with trying to eradicate malaria in many countries; and that the region included "areas inhabited by populations with primitive tribal organizations incapable of supporting complex administrative structures and high costs of malaria eradication campaigns."[8] Many experts in the 1960s believed that malaria in many areas might be eradicated in coming years, but after investments in malaria research and control declined from previous levels and little attention was paid to sub-Saharan Africa, the 1990s saw the resurgence of the disease.

Several high-level meetings and summits have addressed the malaria problem in recent years, reflecting growing political interest in and public recognition of the negative economic and social impacts of malaria on affected regions. For example, in 1995, the U.N. General Assembly expressed concern about malaria's detrimental effects on many developing countries in light of increasing malaria infection rates. The Pan-Africa Malaria Summit of 1997 culminated in the Harare Declaration on Malaria Prevention and Control in the Context of African Economic Recovery and Development. In the Harare Declaration, many African heads of state invited "governments and other partners including multilateral and bilateral agencies to participate actively in a vigorous coordinated effort to control malaria in Africa" and pledged their commitment to the African Plan of Action against malaria described in the declaration. A few years later, many African heads of state agreed to the Abuja Declaration on Roll Back Malaria in Africa, which set targets for reducing malaria's impact in Africa.[9]

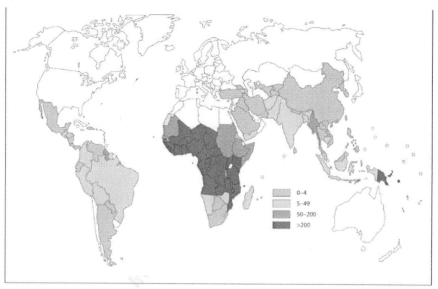

Source: World Health Organization (WHO), World Malaria Report 2008.
Note: Incidence is the rate of occurrence.

Figure 1. Estimated Incidence of Malaria, 2006 per 1,000 population

Since the late 1990s, governments and international organizations have increased public sector investments in malaria control and research, the private sector has contributed funds to new business coalitions against the disease, and renewed coordinating efforts to reach new goals and raise more funding have gotten under way. The World Health Organization (WHO), the U.N. Children's Fund (UNICEF), the U.N. Development Programme (UNDP), and the World Bank launched the Roll Back Malaria Partnership (RBM), a partnership of organizations that aims to provide a coordinated global approach to fighting malaria. The U.N. General Assembly resolved to halt and begin to reverse the incidence of malaria by 2015 as part of the Millennium Development Goals (MDGs). Then the World Health Assembly of WHO urged Member-States to increase financial support and national planning for malaria control.[10]

U.S. EFFORTS TO COMBAT GLOBAL MALARIA

U.S. policymakers have demonstrated strong interest in combating global malaria over the past ten years. Recognizing the global impact of malaria and its relationship to global HIV/AIDS and tuberculosis challenges, Congress provided increased malaria funding for FY200 1 through FY2008 through the Assistance for International Malaria Control Act of 2000 (Control Act, P.L. 106-570) and the United States Leadership Against HIV/AIDS, Tuberculosis, and Malaria Act of 2003 (Leadership Act, P.L. 108-25).[11] However, in 2004 and 2005, criticism of U.S. global malaria policies grew among global health experts and other observers. Some Members of Congress also questioned the U.S. strategy for fighting global malaria, holding congressional hearings to examine USAID's malaria policies and introducing legislation to change the coordination, planning, and spending priorities of U.S. malaria efforts. [12] They expressed concern that USAID 's malaria programs focused mainly on technical assistance rather than purchasing and distributing commodities, such as antimalarial drugs and ITNs, and that malaria activities sometimes did not utilize effective interventions to fight the disease. Some also suggested that the agency was either unable or unwilling to provide requested information about programs' results and spending on malaria interventions and that U.S. malaria efforts might be ineffective. One Member noted that recent increases in funding for U.S. malaria activities coincided with a 10% increase in malaria-related deaths in Africa.[13] At the time, USAID spent almost 8% of its FY2004 malaria budget and almost 10% of its FY2005 malaria budget on commodities.[14]

In 2005, U.S. policymakers tried to address such concerns and criticisms through several key changes to the policies and structure of U.S. malaria programs. USAID reorganized its malaria programs and altered its malaria policies to emphasize funding for procuring commodities and their effective distribution and implementation, program transparency, and monitoring and evaluation activities.[15] That year, President George W. Bush also proposed the President's Malaria Initiative (PMI), a five-year initiative to halve the number of malaria-related deaths in 15 sub- Saharan African countries by 2010, and pledged an additional $1.2 billion over the five years for U.S. global malaria programs through PMI.[16] Some suggest the initiative was part of the Bush Administration's broader African development agenda, which sought to address poverty and disease, among other things, in sub-Saharan Africa. President Bush announced PMI the week before the 2005 G-8 Summit, which had Africa's development as one of its themes; during the Summit, President Bush urged other donors to increase support for malaria efforts in Africa. Although USAID operated malaria programs in many countries before these policy and program changes, these shifts led USAID to concentrate its malaria resources in fewer countries and regions, beginning in 2006.[17] The agency also reported that its intention was to "combine all malaria activities into a single, strategic, global malaria program."[18] Some suggest that PMI is the model for this effort and that, in time, PMI and non-PMI malaria programs may be combined under a broader U.S. malaria program.[19]

After the launch of PMI, Congress continued to express strong interest in U.S. efforts to combat global malaria. During a 2006 congressional hearing on U.S. malaria efforts that evaluated the changes in U.S. global malaria policy and programs, some Members applauded the creation and rapid implementation of the PMI approach in several countries but discussed the need for continued improvement in U.S. malaria activities.[20] In 2008, Congress passed the Tom Lantos and Henry J. Hyde United States Global Leadership Against HIV/AIDS, Tuberculosis, and Malaria Reauthorization Act (Lantos-Hyde Act, P.L. 110-293), which authorizes $5 billion from FY2009 through FY2013 for U.S. global malaria efforts.[21] It also directs the U.S. President to develop a comprehensive, five-year U.S. government strategy to fight global malaria and authorizes the position of a Coordinator of U.S. Government Activities to Combat Malaria Globally (U.S. Global Malaria Coordinator).

During the 2008 Presidential campaign, then Senator Barack Obama pledged to make the United States a global leader in ending malaria-related deaths by 2015.[22] The Obama Administration has stated that it "will continue to build on its commitment to save lives through increasing investments in global health programs ... while also emphasizing a commitment to HIV/AIDS, malaria, and tuberculosis through successful programs, such as PEPFAR and the Malaria Initiative."[23] It is unclear, however, whether the Administration plans to continue PMI's focus on 15 countries or instead adopt an approach that eliminates distinctions between PMI and non-PMI countries. Similarly, while Members of Congress have stated support for U.S. global malaria programs, Congress has not specified that certain countries should be targeted by U.S. malaria efforts, and some suggest that by authorizing the broader role of a U.S. Global Malaria Coordinator instead of the position of the PMI Coordinator, Congress indicated support for a more integrated U.S. approach to global malaria.

U.S. Global Malaria Coordinator

The U.S. Global Malaria Coordinator at USAID oversees and coordinates all U.S. government activities to fight malaria globally, including U.S. global malaria efforts in not only the 15 PMI countries in sub-Saharan Africa but also in other countries and regions that are not part of PMI. Initially, the 2005 creation of PMI brought selected USAID malaria country programs under the oversight of the PMI Coordinator. Through the Lantos-Hyde Act, however, Congress authorized the U.S. Global Malaria Coordinator position, outlining a broader role. This, in effect, replaced the PMI Coordinator with the U.S. Global Malaria Coordinator position.

An Interagency Steering Group advises the U.S. Global Malaria Coordinator and is made up of representatives of USAID, the Department of Health and Human Services, the Department of

State, the Department of Defense, the National Security Council, and the Office of Management and Budget.

U.S. Programs to Fight Global Malaria

USAID and CDC are the primary U.S. agencies that carry out programs to fight malaria globally. USAID supports malaria programs in a number of countries, which may be divided into two groups. The first group consists of 15 countries in sub-Saharan Africa that are part of PMI. The second group consists of countries and regions that are not part of PMI but in which USAID carries out programs to fight malaria. These efforts complement USAID's central programs that address malaria, which are carried out by USAID's Africa Bureau and Global Health Bureau. CDC also carries out operational and applied malaria research and provides technical assistance to U.S. malaria programs or foreign Ministries of Health in a number of countries, including PMI countries, through its Malaria Branch. The U.S. government also contributes to multilateral efforts to fight malaria through not only financial support but also through project coordination and technical assistance to partners' efforts.

President's Malaria Initiative[24]

PMI is the coordinated U.S. government effort to fight malaria in 15 sub-Saharan African countries with high malaria rates: Angola, Benin, Ethiopia, Ghana, Kenya, Liberia, Madagascar, Malawi, Mali, Mozambique, Rwanda, Senegal, Tanzania, Uganda, and Zambia. PMI is led by USAID and implemented by USAID in conjunction with CDC.

The U.S. Global Malaria Coordinator and the Interagency Steering Group selected the 15 PMI countries based on several factors, including whether a country had high rates of malaria, malaria control policies that were in line with internationally accepted standards, the ability to carry out these policies; and a willingness to work with the U.S. government to fight malaria. In the past, after a country was designated a PMI country, the PMI Coordinator would oversee the ongoing USAID malaria program in that country; now PMI country programs are overseen by the U.S. Global Malaria Coordinator.

Over three fiscal years, PMI's implementing agencies expanded PMI's activities to these 15 countries (see Figure 2 for when a country's inclusion in PMI was announced). In FY2006, PMI began operations in the three initial countries – Angola, Tanzania, and Uganda, using some of USAID's FY2005 malaria funding to launch its activities. In FY2007, it added four countries – Malawi, Mozambique, Rwanda, and Senegal, and in FY2008 it added another eight countries – Benin, Ethiopia (Oromiya region), Ghana, Kenya, Liberia, Madagascar, Mali, and Zambia.

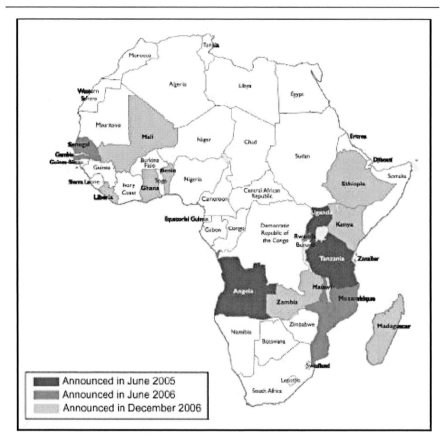

Source: PMI, *Progress Through Partnerships: Saving Lives in Africa*, Second Annual
    Report, March 2008.
Note: In Ethiopia, only one region (Oromiya) was selected for PMI support.

Figure 2. President's Malaria Initiative Countries.

In these 15 countries, the main target of the PMI program is to reach 85%
of those most vulnerable to malaria — children under five years of age and
pregnant women — with a package of four prevention and treatment
measures: treatment using ACTs; IPTp; IRS; and ITNs.[25]

Commodities
Part of the PMI strategy has been to significantly increase spending on the
procurement of commodities above pre-PMI levels.[26] However, PMI
programs' support for specific commodities varies by country due to the
contributions of other donors.

The PMI program supports the procurement of ACTs for the treatment of uncomplicated malaria.[27] As of January 2008, PMI reports that it has procured more than 12.7 million ACT treatments, of which more than 7.4 million have already been distributed to health facilities.

PMI efforts are often integrated with maternal and child health services as part of a package of health interventions to promote mother and infant health. These integrated programs provide pregnant women with a variety of commodities, such as ITNs, as well as health services and treatments, such as IPTp and immunizations, over the course of one or more visits to the doctor.[28] As of January 2008, PMI implementing agencies report that they have procured more than 1.35 million treatments of IPTp, of which more than 583,000 have been distributed to health facilities.

To deliver free or low-cost ITNs to the poorest and most vulnerable groups, PMI implementing agencies often partner with national governments and other organizations and donors in mass campaigns to distribute these commodities. These mass campaigns focus on child survival and may also include vaccination against measles or polio, Vitamin A supplementation, treatment for intestinal worms, and other maternal and child health interventions. PMI efforts also utilize existing programs (such as the maternal and child health efforts described above) to deliver nets. Most PMI-funded ITNs are provided free to vulnerable populations, but in countries where the policy is not to provide free nets, PMI may subsidize the cost of purchase or promote the commercial sale of nets. The PMI program prefers to procure and distribute LLINs, which are longer-lasting ITNs, and also aims to educate users about not only the benefits of ITNs but also their correct use. As of January 2008, PMI implementing agencies report that they have procured more than 6 million LLINs, two-thirds of which have been distributed; re-treated more than 1.1 million ITNs; and procured and distributed an additional 875,000 re-treatment kits.

To complement consistent, correct use of ITNs, PMI programs support the use of IRS as an additional method of mosquito control. In addition to educating local residents about IRS, PMI country programs often provide a supply of insecticide, which is selected based on local malaria conditions from a list of 12 WHO-approved insecticides, and train local personnel on its correct application. As of January 2008, PMI implementing agencies report that their programs in 10 of its 15 PMI countries have carried out IRS of homes, benefiting more than 17 million people.

National Malaria Control Programs

Part of the PMI approach is a "commitment to strengthen national malaria control programs [NMCPs] and to build capacity for eventual country ownership of malaria control efforts."[29] USAID cooperates with the NMCP of each PMI country's government by working within the overall strategy and plan of the country's NMCP. USAID asserts that PMI programs contribute to capacity building of NMCPs in the areas of pharmaceutical management, malaria diagnosis, IRS, malaria in pregnancy, and monitoring and evaluation. More broadly, as a part of procuring and distributing the commodities described above, PMI programs also address underlying capacity issues in PMI countries. As of January 2008, PMI implementing agencies reported that their programs had trained more than 29,000 health workers in the correct use of ACTs and more than 5,000 health workers in how to administer IPTp treatments.

Partners

PMI efforts sometimes operate alongside other U.S. global health efforts, including programs of the President's Emergency Plan for AIDS Relief (PEPFAR). PEPFAR is the coordinated U.S. effort to fight HIV/AIDS globally. The Office of the Global AIDS Coordinator (OGAC) in the Department of State oversees PEPFAR programs, which operate in a number of U.S. agencies.[30] PEPFAR programs also operate in 7 of the 15 countries in which PMI programs exist.[31] In these countries, PMI and PEPFAR staff cooperate on complementary efforts and share mechanisms for commodity delivery when possible.

In carrying out PMI activities, PMI implementing agencies partner with a number of multilateral organizations including the Global Fund to Fight AIDS, Tuberculosis, and Malaria (Global Fund); WHO; RBM; the World Bank; and UNICEF.[32] It also works with the private sector as well as non-governmental organizations (NGOs), including faith-based organizations (FBOs) and community-based organizations (CBOs). Some of these non-governmental organizations may help to expand PMI's reach through the Malaria Communities Program (MCP), a PMI program that funds efforts to fight malaria through NGOs that have not previously partnered with the U.S. government.[33]

Other USAID Malaria Programs[34]

As USAID has scaled-up its PMI activities in the 15 PMI countries, it has also re-evaluated its malaria programs in other countries, eliminating some altogether while concentrating resources in the remainder, in order to "implement programs on a scale that can achieve demonstrable results." In addition to its programs in PMI countries, USAID currently conducts anti-malaria programs in three other countries in Africa — the Democratic Republic of Congo, Nigeria, and southern Sudan. It also supports two regional programs, which are primarily focused on identifying and containing antimalarial drug resistance. These are the Mekong Regional Initiative, which operates in Cambodia, Laos, Thailand, and Vietnam, and the Amazon Initiative, which operates in Brazil, Bolivia, Colombia, Ecuador, Guyana, Peru, and Suriname. Additionally, USAID sometimes provides one-time assistance and humanitarian assistance (through the provision of commodities to fight malaria) to selected countries that would not otherwise receive malaria funding through USAID programs. It provided one-time assistance to Sao Tome and Principe in FY2008 and humanitarian assistance to Zimbabwe in FY2009.

The strategies used in USAID's malaria programs in these non-PMI countries vary depending on the country's malaria situation, national malaria policy, and the contributions of other partners. For example, in Nigeria, USAID reports that it supported the sale of more than 3.5 million ITNs. Another example is the Amazon Initiative: in this region, USAID focused its efforts on the adoption of ACTs as the initial malaria therapy and assisted countries with a variety of issues, including mosquito control, standardized approaches to monitoring resistance, and evaluating the impact of malaria in pregnancy.

CDC Malaria Activities[35]

CDC reports that over the past three decades it has played a role in helping to develop and evaluate malaria prevention and control tools, including ITNs, IPTp, and ACTs, through its operations and applied research. For example, in cooperation with partners, CDC has played a role in studying the impact of malaria during pregnancy in sub-Saharan Africa and helped to develop and evaluate IPTp as a prevention strategy. CDC is also conducting similar work in Latin America. In Kenya, CDC supports a research station that conducts malaria field and laboratory research, disease surveillance, program support through technical assistance, and capacity development through training of Kenyan colleagues. CDC also supports other countries' malaria research efforts through technical assistance and collaboration, as it does in India.

In addition to PMI countries, CDC provides technical assistance to USAID malaria programs and to foreign Ministries of Health in malaria endemic countries that are not part of PMI. In the 15 PMI countries in sub-Saharan Africa, CDC provides technical assistance in program design, implementation, and monitoring and evaluation; and conducts operations research to identify and fill knowledge gaps.[36] For example, in Malawi, the CDC staff focus on strengthening the NMCP by helping to develop national malaria policies and guidelines. In Tanzania, CDC staff collaborate with the Ifakara Health Research and Development Centre on implementation and applied research, which helps to guide malaria control programs in Tanzania as well as other countries in sub-Saharan Africa. CDC's Malaria Branch will soon have staff placed in all 15 PMI countries as technical advisors on the PMI country team. It also provides technical assistance, especially focused on antimalarial drug resistance, to the two USAID regional initiatives in the Amazon and Mekong river basins. CDC staff may be detailed to USAID to support malaria programs at the regional levels. In addition to its role in PMI, CDC provides technical assistance in other countries that have high malaria infection rates, most recently in Indonesia, India, Equatorial Guinea, the Democratic Republic of Congo, Haiti, and Burkina-Faso.

Internationally, CDC works with multilateral partners such as the Global Fund, RBM, UNICEF, WHO, and the World Bank. In some cases, CDC staff are detailed to these partner organizations to provide expertise on a variety of issues, including policy development, program guidance and support, and monitoring and evaluation of progress toward international malaria goals.[37]

Funding

The 2008 Lantos-Hyde Act (P.L. 110-293) authorizes $5 billion for U.S. global efforts to combat malaria from FY2009 through FY2013. It also authorizes up to $2 billion for U.S. contributions to the Global Fund to Fight AIDS, Tuberculosis, and Malaria (Global Fund) in FY2009 and such sums as may be necessary from FY20 10 through FY2013.

Table 1. Funding for U.S. Global Malaria Programs, FY2004 through FY2009 Current U.S. $ Millions

Malaria Program	FY2004 Actual	FY2005 Actual	FY2006 Actual	FY2007 Actual	FY2008 Actual	FY04-FY08 Total	FY2009 Enacted
USAID	79.9	90.8	102.0	248.0	349.6	870.3	382.5[a]
Of which, PMI	*n/a*	*4.3*	*30.0*	*154.2*	*296.0*	*484.5*	
CDC	9.2	9.1	9.0	8.9	8.7	44.9	9.4[a]
Total	**89.1**	**99.9**	**111.0**	**256.9**	**358.3**	**915.2**	**391.9**

Source: Prepared by the Congressional Research Service (CRS) from correspondence with agency officials; PMI, *Saving the Lives of Mothers and Children in Africa*, First Annual Report, March 2007; data provided to CRS by USAID, "FY2006-FY2008 Malaria Budgets," October 7, 2008; congressional budget justifications; and FY2009 Omnibus Appropriations Act (P.L. 111-8), and its accompanying Joint Explanatory Statement.

Note: "n/a" means not applicable. "n/s" means not specified.

a. Specified in the Joint Explanatory Statement.

From FY2004 through FY2008, USAID and CDC received more than $915 million for U.S. efforts to fight global malaria (**Table 1**). Of this, more than $484 million was directed to the President's Malaria Initiative from FY2005 through FY2008.[38] For FY2009, Congress has appropriated $391.9 million for U.S. global malaria programs.

From FY2004 through FY2008, the U.S. government provided $3 billion for U.S. contributions to the Global Fund (**Table 2**). For FY2009, Congress has appropriated $900 million for U.S. contributions to the Global Fund. Although Congress cannot direct the Global Fund to allot specific amounts of the U.S. contribution to projects aimed at a particular disease, the Global Fund reports that it awarded the following percentages of all contributions to malaria projects: 31% during round 4, 27% during round 5, 24% during round 6, and 25% during round 7.[39]

POLICY ISSUES

When considering U.S. efforts to address malaria, Members of the 111th Congress may wish to take a number of issues into account.[40]

Table 2. U.S. Contributions to the Global Fund, FY2004 through FY2009
Current U.S. $ Millions

Agency	FY2004 Actual	FY2005 Actual	FY2006 Actual	FY2007 Actual	FY2008 Actual	FY04-FY08 Total	FY2009 Enacted
USAID	397.6	248.0	247.5	247.5	0.0	1140.6	0.1
FY2004 Carryover[a]	(87.8)	87.8	n/a	n/a	n/a	n/a	n/a
State	0.0	0.0	198.0	377.5	545.5	1121.0	600.0
NIH	149.1	99.2	99.0	99.0	294.8	741.1	300.0
Total	**458.9**	**435.0**	**544.5**	**724.0**	**840.3**	**3,002.7**	**900.0**

Source: Prepared by CRS from congressional budget justifications; correspondence with agency officials; FY2009 Omnibus Appropriations Act (P.L. 111-8) and its accompanying Joint Explanatory Statement; and CRS Report RL33485, *U.S. International HIV/AIDS, Tuberculosis, and Malaria Spending: FY2004-FY2008*, by Tiaji SalaamBlyther.

Note: The Department of State portion of the contribution was from the Global HIV/AIDS Initiative (GHAI) account, which is now included in the Global Health and Child Survival (GHCS) account.

a. In FY2004, $87.8 million of U.S. contributions to the Global Fund was withheld per legislative provision that prohibit U.S. contributions to the Fund to exceed 33% of all contributions. The FY2005 Consolidated Appropriations Act released these funds to the Global Fund, subject to the 33% proviso.

PMI Structure and Scope

Some malaria experts question whether the PMI structure is sustainable. A key concern is whether key distinctions between PMI and non-PMI country programs will persist, especially the disparity between PMI and non-PMI programs in resources. This, some malaria experts maintain, is not a sustainable approach to fighting malaria in Africa, because it does not recognize that progress in PMI countries may be reversed if malaria is not also controlled in non-PMI countries that have high rates of malaria, in light of the movement of people across borders and disease transmission patterns within regions. They argue that the PMI country selection process excluded countries with more complex malaria problems that may have required greater resources and where many malaria infections and deaths occur, limiting the U.S. response to malaria in these places. However, others assert that excluding such countries allowed more resources to be spent in countries with fewer program implementation and funding distribution challenges. As a result, implementing partners in selected PMI countries may have been able to progress more quickly in targeted areas and, through these experiences, learn best practices that might be brought to scale in non-PMI countries with additional resources and funding. Advocates recommend that Congress ensure that the five-year U.S. strategy to address global malaria, which Congress directed the Administration to develop in the Lantos-Hyde Act, addresses these issues.

Advocates urge Congress to expand PMI's scope to include additional countries. Supporters of PMI expansion maintain that non-PMI countries with high malaria infection and mortality rates, such as the Democratic Republic of Congo, Nigeria, and southern Sudan, would benefit from increased funding and resources. These proponents assert that PMI is a successful model for other bilateral malaria initiatives and that PMI has demonstrated measurable results that show improvements in malaria mortality rates. They contend that PMI has been successful, because implementing partners have applied many of the lessons learned from implementing PEPFAR to PMI programs. For example, PMI implementing partners have replicated PEPFAR processes such as having one country coordinator who oversees all projects and ensures that all initiatives utilize a common strategy in their execution; collaborating on program implementation and budget planning; concentrating resources on commodity procurement and distribution; and, to the extent possible, coordinating its efforts with other U.S. maternal and child health interventions. Even if the number of PMI countries is not increased, some who support expansion argue that Congress should extend the related mandates and strategies of PMI to countries with high malaria rates.

Critics of PMI expansion often agree with proponents that PMI is a model for other bilateral malaria efforts and that its approach to fighting malaria may shape the five-year U.S. global malaria strategy. However, PMI expansion opponents contend that PMI should remain limited to the current 15 countries to preserve and support progress toward the five-year targets in each country. They assert that expanding the initiative may distract from the public impact of successful ongoing efforts, which has positive effects for U.S. public diplomacy efforts and also increases recipient country support for U.S. malaria programs. One argument made by those with this view is that including countries with more complex malaria problems and much larger populations would require significant increases in PMI funding and extend U.S. commitments to recipient countries.

Funding for U.S. Malaria Programs

Some advocates urge Congress to increase funding for U.S. malaria programs to reach the Lantos-Hyde Act authorized level of $5 billion from FY2009 through FY2013. This would allow PMI's implementing agencies to extend coverage to more areas; purchase and distribute more commodities; and expand access to related services, such as malaria education and technical assistance. Some malaria experts caution against reducing malaria funding. Supporters of higher PMI funding maintain that decreased support for ongoing U.S. malaria efforts might lead to drug and parasite resistance and threaten advancements made in controlling malaria in areas where U.S. programs have expanded access to key malaria commodities that control the disease.

In the absence of increased funding for U.S. malaria programs, many observers advocate maintaining current funding levels to preserve improvements in malaria control in PMI countries and to allow U.S. malaria programs to continue ongoing programs. However, if U.S. malaria programs were not able to realize greater cost efficiencies in purchasing and distributing commodities and other activities, current levels of funding would not allow programs to expand. One argument made by opponents to increasing PMI funding is that support might reduce available funding for other U.S. global health efforts. Over the past five years, funding for U.S. global malaria activities has grown considerably, while other activities, such as child survival and maternal health (CS/MH) and family planning and reproductive health programs (FP/RH), have received small increases in funding.[41] Others, however, argue that malaria efforts were previously underfunded and that increased funding during this period reflects the U.S. commitment to adequately funding malaria activities and still remains less than CS/MH and FP/RH funding levels.

Some health experts assert that the debate about whether increases in support for U.S. malaria programs, especially PMI, come at the expense of other global health programs exists because overall U.S. global health funding is insufficient. This view holds that U.S. global health programs are inadequately funded relative to the challenges posed to global health by not only infectious diseases like malaria but also other issues such as chronic diseases, climate change, hunger, urbanization, and clean water and sanitation. Opponents of this view agree that global health challenges are considerable but assert that they cannot be addressed by U.S. bilateral programs alone; they contend that leveraging current funding through coordination and collaboration with other governments' and multilateral malaria efforts is a better approach to resource and funding constraints. Some of these critics also maintain that malaria funding, like other U.S. global health funding, should not be increased in light of U.S. budgetary constraints, the conflicts in Iraq and Afghanistan, and other issues.

Reporting on U.S. Malaria Funding and Activities

Some health and malaria experts assert that PMI does not disburse funds quickly enough, which may slow the scale-up of malaria programs and limit the efforts of partners that rely on USAID funding. Other critics argue that PMI should be required to publicly report PMI funding disbursements in addition to the currently reported committed or planned amounts. They assert that it is difficult to evaluate the effectiveness of efforts without knowing how quickly funding reaches recipients.

Those advocating for stronger PMI reporting and transparency requirements also contend that with the increased authority of the U.S. Global Malaria Coordinator, the more stringent standard of transparency and detail in reporting that has been applied to PMI countries' activities should be expanded to USAID malaria programs in other areas. One argument made by these observers is that since the reorganization of some of these activities under PMI, public reporting of objectives and achievements in USAID's malaria programs outside of the 15 PMI countries has become less detailed and is often limited to overall malaria country and regional project budgets. Another argument made by some is that CDC's role in U.S. malaria efforts, especially in the area of technical assistance should be clearly and distinctly described in reports on U.S. global efforts to fight malaria, including the annual PMI report. Other experts assert that Congress should direct the Administration to address malaria challenges in non-PMI countries and regions, such as the Democratic Republic of Congo, Nigeria, and southern Sudan, in the new U.S. global malaria strategy.

Balance between Commodities and Technical Assistance

Some experts argue that while PMI has increased the amount of funding available for commodities, the balance between providing commodities and technical assistance should be examined. Some malaria authorities assert that technical assistance is key to the design and sustainability of effective malaria control programs in countries with weak health infrastructures. While many such countries now receive greater funding for malaria control activities and donors often allow their funding to be spent on purchasing and distributing commodities, malaria experts point out that fewer donors support technical assistance. These experts maintain that the development of local knowledge of how to manage malaria will be key to preventing the disease from resurging as it has in the past when outside funding and international attention waned.

Other health professionals question whether increased funding for technical assistance efforts is prudent. They express concern about the cost of consultants and question whether money is better used to support commodities that are sometimes in short supply or out of reach for the most vulnerable populations. Those that make this argument suggest that, as in USAID's pre-PMI malaria efforts, focusing on technical assistance instead of providing commodities does not give countries the health interventions and commodities necessary to reduce malaria infection rates and deaths.[42]

Still, some malaria experts say that it is not a choice between commodities and technical assistance: they believe that comprehensive efforts to address malaria through U.S. programs should address both. They assert that while past efforts that focused on technical assistance without commodities did not produce significant results, today the contributions of many donors and national governments to global malaria efforts and funding might allow some programs to focus more on technical assistance while others emphasize funding for commodities.

Commodities: Accessibility and Affordability

Malaria experts and global health groups debate how the United States can best provide access to life-saving commodities in countries where there are high rates of malaria infection: through free or subsidized commodities or through market channels. Some health experts argue that the United States should ensure access and effectiveness of commodities by either subsidizing commodity prices or providing them for free. In the case of antimalarial drugs, for example, in 2004 the Institute of Medicine and other groups recommended that governments and international organizations subsidize the global market for ACTs.[43] At the time, ACTs cost about 10 times as much as the most frequently used drug at the time, chloroquine, which was becoming increasingly ineffective due to parasite resistance. Proponents say that subsidizing antimalarial drugs would help make them more widely available, decrease their prices, and, with accurate and quick diagnosis, delay the emergence of parasite resistance to antimalarial drugs.[44] Proponents of subsidizing other malaria commodities, such as ITNs and RDTs, make similar arguments.

However, opponents believe that malaria commodities should be provided for free in areas with high rates of malaria, because in these regions, many people often live in poverty and cannot afford the cost — even at a subsidized price — of drugs or insecticide-treated nets. One of the arguments opponents make is that providing free tools for preventing, diagnosing, and treating malaria would ensure access for the poor and protect health in the broader community by aiding, for example, the accurate and prompt use of effective antimalarial drugs or the use of ITNs, which both help to reduce malaria transmission community-wide. On the other hand, opponents of free nets contend that U.S. malaria efforts should support countries' capacities to either produce or purchase commodities through the private sector. For example, they believe ITNs should be provided through market channels, because they are concerned that giving away nets may undermine the market for them. One argument opponents of free nets make is that free nets may not be valued by recipients to the degree that purchased nets would be. They express concern that free nets would be used incorrectly or inconsistently compared to those bought at regular or even lower subsidized prices.

In addition to debates about pricing commodities for consumers, health experts and NGOs point out that the high demand for commodities created by donor programs, such as PMI and other donors' malaria programs, has led to supply shortages. Despite growing demand from programs like PMI, demand for these commodities from potential recipients is often not as high, due to a lack of education about malaria and the benefits of using these commodities as well as an inability to pay for them. In many malaria endemic countries for a number of reasons — including few commodity producers, high start-up costs, and low profit margins — lack of sufficient commodity production capacity and supply persists, sometimes leading to "stock-outs," which is when malaria programs do not have adequate commodities on hand to carry out their activities. In the absence of additional producers entering these markets, some experts assert that without the involvement of initiatives such as PMI, which may negotiate for large orders of commodities, existing producers may be wary of increasing capacity without knowing that commodities will be purchased at a reasonable price at a particular time.

Some health and development experts recommend that donors and national governments address not only issues related to commodity supplies but also focus on commodity procurement and supply chain management to ensure that needed commodities are accurately forecast. They point out that better procurement and supply chain management would not only improve donors' efforts to negotiate for sufficient supplies and commodity industries' plans for production but also prevent stock-outs and the expiration of commodities before they can be bought and distributed. Other experts express concern that some producers may not feel that the low negotiated prices for some commodities make additional investments sufficiently profitable to increase production to meet forecasted commodity needs and suggest that perhaps commodity production should also be subsidized, either directly or through price floors for commodity producers, or made more attractive through incentives, such as tax breaks.

Commodities: Effectiveness

Concerns about how effective commodities may be are closely related to their accessibility and availability: as commodities to address malaria have become more widespread in recent years, parasite and mosquito resistance and misdiagnosis of malaria have become greater problems, impacting how effective or ineffective current commodities are. In some parts of the world, parasite resistance to some malaria medications and mosquito resistance to insecticides are increasing due to several factors, including varying degrees of accessibility or availability of commodities. Drug ineffectiveness has been a problem in past efforts to fight malaria when malaria parasites became increasingly resistant to commonly-used drugs such as chloroquine. An increase in parasite resistance to ACTs in some regions (particularly along the Thai-Cambodian border) has led many experts, including those at WHO, to express concern. Since chloroquine resistance was first noticed in this same area, experts worry that without careful attention to efforts to prevent misuse of ACTs, ACTs will become ineffective before an equally effective alternative antimalarial drug is available. Parasite resistance to SP is also a growing problem.[45] Also contributing to the increase in drug-resistant malaria and, therefore, the risk of drug ineffectiveness is misdiagnosis of malaria or misuse of drugs and other commodities, where available. Misdiagnosis may be the result of several factors, including the difficulty of distinguishing between malaria and other diseases with similar symptoms when a lack of laboratory facilities or accurate, quick diagnostic tools (such as rapid diagnostic tests (RDTs)) exists in an area. RDTs allow healthcare workers to more accurately diagnose malaria, because the tests require only a drop of blood and 15 minutes before the results are known. Malaria previously could only be confirmed through laboratory tests that are not readily available in many malaria-endemic areas. While PMI programs procured 505,000 RDTs and distributed 101,000 of them as of January 2008, health experts recommend that malaria programs increase the number of RDTs available and distribute them more widely.[46]

As drug and mosquito resistance to commonly used malaria commodities increases, many malaria experts maintain that malaria programs should not only address misuse of malaria commodities through education but also that donors and national governments should make greater investments in research and development of alternatives to current drugs and insecticides. Malaria experts emphasize that to limit the growth of resistance, donors and national governments' malaria programs need to address incorrect use of commodities through education and ensure that coverage with key malaria interventions continues to increase, especially in areas with high rates of malaria where the entire community benefits from high levels of ITN and IRS use. These experts also express concern that despite the possibility that current malaria drugs and insecticides may one day become ineffective due to resistance, the number of new drugs and insecticides being developed to prevent and treat malaria has declined in recent years.[47] They urge donors and national governments to invest in such research so that alternatives will be available when resistance increases, as it already is in some areas.

Many experts and policymakers express concern about the negative impact of counterfeit or low quality antimalarial drugs on the effective, safe treatment of malaria. Health authorities report that counterfeit and substandard antimalarials threaten not only the health of infected individuals — who believe they are receiving treatment but actually are not — but also the health of their communities. They assert that ineffective malaria treatment undermines trust in malaria treatment programs and regimens and also allows the malaria parasite to persist, which increases the possibility of further transmission of malaria within the community and may contribute to greater drug resistance. These health professionals recommend that national and international authorities create and enforce strategies to prevent the production, sale, trade, and use of counterfeit or low quality medicines.[48]

Some debate surrounds the use of certain insecticides, especially dichlorodiphenyltrichloroethane (DDT), by malaria control programs, including U.S. programs. Some environmental groups express concern about the possible impact of insecticides, particularly DDT, on the environment and on human health, arguing that these compounds may stay in the environment for years after their initial use and might enter the food chain. However, some malaria experts maintain that the amount of insecticides used for indoor residual spraying is a small fraction of the amount of insecticide used in agriculture. These malaria professionals contend that the risks to human health of not effectively controlling the population of mosquitoes that transmit malaria are greater than the potential risk to human health of using some insecticides. Some trade and development experts observe that insecticide use may negatively impact developing countries' trade relationships with other countries and regions, such as the European Union (EU), because of recent restrictions on the use of certain insecticides. Health experts, however, raise questions about the possible negative impact of such restrictions on the availability, affordability, and use of insecticides for public health purposes.[49] These health authorities suggest that donors and governments should support the market for public health insecticides (PHIs) by investing in research and development of new insecticides and promoting the use of effective insecticides for IRS and ITNs.

Disease-Specific versus Health Systems Approach

Some observers oppose a disease-specific approach to global health such as that taken by PMI, which they argue focuses too narrowly on only one disease. They maintain that such an approach ignores the interconnected nature of health care challenges and diverts resources from other health efforts.[50] They argue that in resource-poor countries, it could create competition for limited workforce capacity such as physicians, public health specialists, and U.S. program managers. Some experts argue that the United States must tackle the underlying weaknesses of many health systems in PMI-assisted areas, such as the lack of hospital and clinic infrastructure, laboratory facilities, and trained healthcare workers. They point out that the budgets of Ministries of Health in many PMI-designated countries are dwarfed by donor funding for disease-specific initiatives like malaria and that much of these Ministries of Health budgets often come from donor sources.[51] This raises two questions, they argue, about the sustainability of disease-specific initiatives. First, are the achievements of disease-specific initiatives sustainable if donor support ends before eradication of a disease? This is especially problematic if

Ministries of Health continue to lack comparable levels of funding or have not developed the expertise required to manage these funds and programs independently. Second, would Ministries of Health prioritize disease-specific efforts in the absence of donor-directed funding? In other words, would they instead prioritize spending on human resources for health, infrastructure improvement, basic health services, and strengthening their countries' health systems in other ways when faced with limited budgets? Disruptions in donor or national government support may lead to reversals in the progress made against diseases like malaria and associated problems, such as increased disease resistance to past prevention and treatment strategies.

However, some health experts support a disease-specific approach. They argue that, in light of the limited resources of many countries facing both weak health systems and high infectious disease burdens, U.S. efforts such as PMI are vital to arresting the deaths from these diseases. Some malaria experts maintain that without sustained, focused attention and donor-directed funding, large-scale eradication of diseases like malaria would be unlikely, as the history of malaria control and eradication has shown. They contend that disease-specific initiatives support the broader health system in which they operate by transmitting knowledge and building platforms through which other health initiatives may grow and cooperate.

Finally, some experts maintain that neither approach would be successful in isolation and assert that directed efforts on specific diseases should occur simultaneously with efforts to build health capacity and infrastructure. While they applaud the initial emphasis of PMI on malaria's prevention and treatment, these observers contend that in light of the authorization of $5 billion for the U.S. global malaria efforts over the next five years, the initiative should further integrate efforts to combat malaria with the provision of basic healthcare and the prevention of childhood illness. Supporters argue that some major donors have already recognized the necessity of both approaches to achieving success in fighting particular diseases. One example is the Global Fund, which provides funding for not only HIV/AIDS, tuberculosis, and malaria projects but also those that focus on strengthening health systems.

PMI and Global Fund Coordination

Some global health observers raise the issue of balance between U.S. malaria funding for bilateral and multilateral malaria efforts. The United States is the largest donor to the Global Fund, which is the leading financier of global malaria programs in the world, yet U.S. funding for bilateral efforts has been growing in recent years. It is unclear whether policymakers are concerned about the balance between U.S. funding directed to multilateral versus bilateral efforts to address malaria. While Congress has expressed strong support for increased bilateral malaria funding in recent years, it has not discussed whether funding for multilateral or bilateral malaria efforts should be examined with perhaps one exception. In 2004-2006, several Members noted during congressional hearings that U.S. bilateral programs did not adequately fund commodity procurement and distribution. Although the Global Fund is not an implementing agency, it does support the purchase and provision of malaria commodities through malaria project grants in many countries. Therefore, in light of subsequent U.S. malaria policy changes that now emphasize funding for commodities, some might argue that policymakers determined that U.S. support for multilateral efforts to provide commodities through the Global Fund were not sufficient and should be complemented by bilateral efforts.

Congress has, however, emphasized the need for coordination to prevent duplication of effort and to leverage funds among partners, which it reiterated in the Lantos-Hyde Act last year. In light of the high levels of funding provided to both bilateral programs, especially PMI, and multilateral efforts to fight malaria, advocates maintain that it is essential for PMI and the Global Fund to coordinate their planning and funding activities. This helps to ensure that funded programs reflect country needs, are not redundant, and operate in a more cost-effective manner. PMI implementing agencies have instituted several processes, based on lessons from PEPFAR, to coordinate PMI programs and funding with the Global Fund. These include cooperating with the Global Fund through NMCPs and other country forums; supporting the development of Global Fund project proposals through these structures; and carrying out joint projects in PMI countries, such as one recent effort in which the Global Fund procured ACTs that the PMI program then distributed. Additionally, U.S. government representatives serve as voting members of the Global Fund Board and on the Board's Policy and Strategy Committee as well its Finance and Audit Committee.[52] However, some malaria experts and global health observers assert that improvement is still needed to ensure that partners' capabilities are reflected in the division of labor in countries, especially with regard to funding technical assistance where other partners, such as the Global Fund, may be able to fund commodities. Others caution that PMI programs should not coordinate efforts to such a degree that the programs' abilities to respond quickly to country needs and reflect U.S. malaria policy priorities might be negatively impacted. Both views urge Congress to examine how U.S. malaria programs leverage their resources and funding in coordinating activities with the Global Fund.

APPENDIX A. ACRONYMS AND ABBREVIATIONS

The table below defines acronyms and abbreviations used in the main body of this report.

Acronyms and Abbreviations

ACTs	Artemisinin-based Combination Therapies
CBOs	Community-Based Organizations
CDC	Centers for Disease Control and Prevention
FBOs	Faith-Based Organizations
Global Fund	Global Fund to Fight AIDS, Tuberculosis, and Malaria
HHS	U.S. Department of Health and Human Services
IPTp	Intermittent Preventive Treatment of Malaria during Pregnancy
IRS	Indoor Residual Spraying
ITNs	Insecticide-Treated Nets
Lantos-Hyde Act	Tom Lantos and Henry J. Hyde United States Global Leadership Against HIV/AIDS, Tuberculosis, and Malaria Reauthorization Act of 2008 (P.L. 110-293)
LLINs	Long-Lasting Insecticidal Nets
MCP	Malaria Communities Program
MDGs	Millennium Development Goals
NGOs	Non-Governmental Organizations
NMCP	National Malaria Control Program
PHIs	Public Health Insecticides
PMI	President's Malaria Initiative
RBM	Roll Back Malaria Partnership
U.N.	United Nations
UNDP	U.N. Development Programme

UNICEF	U.N. Children's Fund
USAID	U.S. Agency for International Development
WHO	World Health Organization

APPENDIX B. SELECTED ADDITIONAL RESOURCES

This section provides a list of selected additional resources on global malaria. Inclusion of a resource in this list should not be interpreted as an endorsement by the Congressional Research Service of ideas presented therein.

Resources

Martin S. Alilio, Ib C. Bygbj erg, & Joel G. Breman. (2004). "Are Multilateral Malaria Research and Control Programs the Most Successful? Lessons from the Past 100 Years in Africa," *The American Journal of Tropical Medicine and Hygiene (AJTMH)*, Vol. *71*, supp. 2, 268- 278.

Roger Bate. (2008). "Rolling Back Malaria: Rhetoric and Reality in the Fight against a Deadly Killer," *Health Policy Outlook*, no. 4, AEI.org, April.

Nicole Bates & James Herrington. (2007). "Advocacy for Malaria Prevention, Control, and Research in the Twenty-First Century," *AJTMH*, Vol. *77*, supp. 6, 314-320.

Luke Gallup & Jeffrey D. Sachs. (2001). "The Economic Burden of Malaria," in *AJTMH*, Vol. *64*, supp. 1, 85–96.

The Lancet, (2006). "The U.S. President's Malaria Initiative," editorial, Vol. *368*, Issue 9523, p. 1, editorial, July 1.

Samuel Loewenberg. (2007). "The U.S. President's Malaria Initiative: 2 Years On," *The Lancet*, Vol. 370, Issue 9603, pp. 1893-1894, December 8.

Randall M. Packard. (2007). *The Making of a Tropical Disease: A Short History of Malaria* (Baltimore: The Johns Hopkins University Press).

WHO. (2001). *Macroeconomics and Health: Investing in Health for Economic Development*, Report of the Commission on Macroeconomics and Health.

APPENDIX C. USAID FUNDING BY PROGRAM

Funding for PMI

Of the $915 million allocated for U.S. global malaria programs from FY2004 through FY2008, over 71% ($619 million) was spent on USAID malaria programs in the 15 countries displayed in **Table C-1**, which are all PMI countries now. A country's malaria funding increased after PMI became operational in it (as indicated by the shaded areas). USAID has allocated the following percentages of total PMI funding in the 15 PMI countries for commodities: 56% in FY2006, 52% in FY2007, 46% in FY2008, and a planned 50% in FY2009.[53]

Table C-1. USAID Funding for Selected Countries and PMI, FY2004 through FY2009 Current U.S. $ Millions

Program	FY2004 Actual	FY2005 Actual	FY2006 Actual	FY2007 Actual	FY2008 Actual	FY04-FY08 Total	FY2009 Planned
Angola	1.0	1.3	7.5	18.5	18.8	47.1	18.7
Benin	2.0	2.0	1.8	3.6	13.9	23.3	13.8
Ethiopia	2.0	2.0	2.6	6.7	19.8	33.1	19.7
Ghana	1.0	1.3	1.5	5.0	16.9	25.7	17.3
Kenya	1.2	1.2	5.5	6.1	19.8	33.8	19.7
Liberia	0.3	0.5	n/a	2.5	12.4	15.7	11.8
Madagascar	2.0	2.3	2.2	5.0	16.9	28.4	16.7
Malawi	1.5	2.1	2.0	18.5	17.9	42.0	17.7
Mali	1.8	2.4	2.5	4.5	14.9	26.1	15.4
Mozambique	1.5	2.1	6.3	18.0	19.8	47.7	19.8
Rwanda	1.0	1.0	1.5	20.0	16.9	40.4	16.3
Senegal	2.5	2.5	2.2	16.7	16.0	39.9	15.7
Tanzania	1.3	1.7	11.5	31.0	33.7	79.2	35.0
Uganda	3.0	3.0	9.5	21.5	21.8	58.8	21.6
Zambia	4.0	4.0	7.7	9.5	14.9	40.1	14.7
PMI Headquarters	n/a	4.3	1.5	10.0	21.6	37.4	n/s
Total	26.1	33.7	65.8	197.1	296.0	618.7	273.9
Of which, PMI	n/a	4.3	30.0	154.2	296.0	484.5	273.9

Source: Prepared by CRS from data presented in PMI, "USAID Malaria Program Inputs FY2004," "Malaria Program Inputs FY2005," "USAID FY2006 CSH Malaria Budgets," http://fightingmalaria.gov/funding data provided to CRS by

USAID, "FY2007 and FY2008 Malaria Budgets," October 7, 2008; and PMI,
"Country Operational Plans,"
http://www.fightingmalaria.gov/countries/mops/index.html, accessed March 17,
2009.

Notes: Shaded areas indicate when PMI became operational in a country. "n/a" means
not available. "n/s" means not specified in funding documents available on PMI
website as of March 17, 2009.

Funding for Other USAID Malaria Programs

Since the creation of PMI, USAID's funding for malaria programs has
shifted from smaller amounts of funding for many countries to greater
amounts for fewer countries and selected regional and central programs (**Table
C-2**). In addition to funding for PMI and central programs through USAID's
Africa and Global Health Bureaus, USAID now supports three non-PMI
country programs and two regional initiatives.

**Table C-2. USAID Funding for Non-PMI Country, Regional, and Central
Malaria Programs, FY2004 through FY2008 Current U.S. $ Millions**

Program	FY2004	FY2005	FY2006	FY2007	FY2008	Total
Burundi	0.5	0.5	---	---	---	1.0
Democratic Republic of Congo (DRC)	2.9	2.1	2.4	6.7	7.2	21.3
DRC FY2005 Carryover	---	0.9	---	---	---	0.9
Eritrea	0.6	0.5	---	---	---	1.1
Eritrea[a]	---	0.3	---	---	---	0.3
Guinea	---	0.3	---	---	---	0.3
Nigeria	2.4	2.9	2.7	6.5	6.9	21.4
Sao Tome and Principe[b]	---	---	---	---	0.5	0.5
Sudan[c]	2.0	2.5	2.0	3.0	4.0	13.5
West Africa Regional	1.5	1.7	---	---	---	3.2
East Africa Regional	2.0	2.1	0.2	---	---	4.3
Africa Regional Bureau	2.6	2.8	1.0	2.0	1.7	10.1
Sub-Saharan Africa Subtotal	**14.5**	**16.6**	**8.3**	**18.2**	**20.3**	**77.9**

Table C-2. (Continued)

Program	FY2004	FY2005	FY2006	FY2007	FY2008	Total
Afghanistan	0.4	1.0	---	---	---	1.4
Burma	0.1	---	---	---	---	0.1
Cambodia	1.4	1.4	1.5	---	---	4.3
India	0.4	0.7	---	---	---	1.1
Indonesia	0.7	1.1	---	---	---	1.8
Nepal	0.7	0.6	---	---	---	1.3
Mekong Regional Initiative	---	---	2.0	5.5	5.5	13.0
Asia and Near East Bureau	2.0	2.0	---	---	---	4.0
Asia Subtotal	**5.7**	**6.8**	**3.5**	**5.5**	**5.5**	**27.0**
Bolivia	0.6	0.8	---	---	---	1.4
Dominican Republic	---	0.5	---	---	---	0.5
Haiti	0.7	1.0	---	---	---	1.7
Honduras	0.3	0.3	---	---	---	0.6
Peru	0.8	0.3	---	---	---	1.1
Amazon Initiative	---	---	2.1	5.0	5.0	12.1
Latin America and the Caribbean (LAC) Regional	1.8	2.1	---	---	---	3.9
LAC Subtotal	**4.2**	**5.0**	**2.1**	**5.0**	**5.0**	**21.3**
Kyrgyzstan	0.1	---	---	---	---	0.1
Tajikistan	0.1	---	---	---	---	0.1
Europe and Eurasia Subtotal	**0.2**	---	---	---	---	**0.2**
Global Health Bureau	29.4	31.7	19.7	22.3	23.0	126.1
Central Programs Subtotal	**29.4**	**31.7**	**19.7**	**22.3**	**23.0**	**126.1**
Total	**54.0**	**60.1**	**33.6**	**51.0**	**53.8**	**252.5**

Source: Prepared by CRS from data presented in PMI, "USAID Malaria Program Inputs FY2004," "Malaria Program Inputs FY2005," "USAID FY2006 CSH Malaria Budgets," http://fightingmalaria.gov/funding data provided to CRS by USAID, "FY2007 and FY2008 Malaria Budgets," October 7, 2008; and CRS Correspondence with Dr. Trent Ruebush, Senior Malaria Advisor, USAID Bureau for Global Health, November 7, 2008.

Notes: Dashes indicate $0 in funding.

a. Not assigned due to mission closure.

b. One-time assistance.

c. Southern Sudan.

APPENDIX D. SELECTED GLOBAL MALARIA PROGRAMS AND ORGANIZATIONS

This section provides a list of selected programs and organizations that address global malaria, including bilateral and multilateral efforts to fight malaria. It also includes private-public partnerships, non-governmental organizations, international alliances, and a coalition of private industry. It provides a brief description of each entity, which is drawn from each organization's website. The programs and organizations listed in this section were randomly selected; their selection should not be interpreted as an endorsement by the Congressional Research Service.

U.S. Government Programs

- Centers for Disease Control and Prevention (CDC) Global Malaria Program, http://www.cdc.gov/malaria
  CDC participates actively in global efforts against malaria through its Global Malaria Program and its role in PMI. Its work spans the spectrum of policy development, program guidance and support, scientific research, monitoring and evaluation of progress toward RBM goals, and technical assistance. It works in malaria-endemic countries with the Ministry of Health and local disease prevention and control partners, in malaria-endemic regional settings, and with key multilateral and bilateral Roll Back Malaria (RBM) partners.
- United States Agency for International Development (USAID) President's Malaria Initiative (PMI), http://fightingmalaria.gov/ or http://www.pmi.gov/.
  PMI represents an historic five-year expansion of U.S. resources to fight malaria in the region most affected by the disease. In 2005, President Bush committed an additional $1.2 billion in malaria funding to PMI with the goal of reducing malaria-related deaths by 50% in 15 countries in sub-Saharan Africa by 2010. PMI is an interagency initiative led by USAID and implemented together with CDC.

Other Organizations

- Affordable Medicines Facility-malaria (AMFm) Taskforce, http :// www.rbm. who. int/globalsubsidytaskforce.html.
  AMFm is an initiative to increase access to effective malaria treatment for people in endemic countries by making ACTs available at a much lower price, so more people will be able to afford them. Initiated in 2007, the AMFm Taskforce is a workstream of the RBM Harmonization Working Group.
- Africa Fighting Malaria (AFM), http://www.fightingmalaria. org/.
  Founded in 2000, AFM is a non-profit health advocacy group whose mission is to make malaria control more transparent, responsive and effective. It conducts research into the social and economic aspects of malaria and raises the profile of the disease and the issues surrounding its control in the local and international media. AFM strives to hold public institutions accountable for funding and implementing effective, integrated and country- driven malaria control policies and to promote successful private sector initiatives to control the disease.
- Bill and Melinda Gates Foundation, http://www. gatesfoundation. org/topics/Pages/malaria
  The Gates Foundation works with partners around the world and supports efforts to speed malaria research, expand access to life-saving drugs and prevention methods, and advocate for greater action.
- CORE   Group   Malaria   Working   Group   (MWG), http://www.coregroup.org/working_groups/malaria
  Established in 1997, CORE Group is a membership association of international nongovernmental organizations (NGOs) whose mission is to improve the health and well being of children and women in developing countries through collaborative NGO action and learning. Collectively, CORE Group members work in 180 countries. The MWG supports existing national collaborative partnerships and promotes new partnerships in which NGOs can actively be engaged in national level policy formation and innovative programming to scale up malaria prevention and control. CORE originally stood for "Child Survival Collaborations and Resources Group."
- Drugs for Neglected Diseases initiative (DNDi), http:// www. dndi. org/.
  In 2003, seven organizations from around the world joined forces to establish DNDi.[54] The initiative fosters collaboration both among

developing countries and between developing and developed countries. Its design is a blend of centralized management to give it a clear project-specific focus, and decentralized operations that mimic modern drug companies. DNDi does not conduct research and scientific work to develop drugs itself. Instead, it capitalizes on existing, fragmented R&D capacity, especially in the developing world, and complements it with additional expertise as needed. DNDi has built regional networks of scientists actively involved in the research of new drugs for neglected diseases in Asia, Africa and Latin America.

- FasterCures, http://www.fastercures.org/.
  FasterCures' mission is to identify and implement global solutions to accelerate the process of discovery and clinical development of new therapies for the treatment of deadly and debilitating diseases. It seeks ways to amplify the productivity of the considerable resources and expansive infrastructure dedicated to finding new medical solutions.

- Global Business Coalition on AIDS, TB, and Malaria (GBC), http://www.businessfightsmalaria.org/home/home.php.
  Founded in 2001, GBC mobilizes international business against HIV/AIDS, tuberculosis, and malaria. The organization represents a rapidly expanding alliance of 220 international companies dedicated to combating the world's deadliest epidemics through the business sector's unique skills and expertise. Building on its success with HIV/AIDS, GBC recently added malaria and tuberculosis to its mandate, advocating business action in four key areas: workplace, community involvement, core competency, and advocacy and leadership. GBC is the official focal point of the private sector delegation to the Global Fund to Fight AIDS, Tuberculosis and Malaria.

- Global Fund to Fight AIDS, Tuberculosis, and Malaria, *http://www. theglobalfund.org/en/*.
  The Global Fund is a unique global public/private partnership between governments, civil society, the private sector and affected communities that works in close collaboration with other bilateral and multilateral organizations to supplement existing efforts dealing with the three diseases. Since its creation in 2002, the Global Fund has become the main source of financing for programs to fight AIDS, tuberculosis and malaria. It provides a quarter of all international

financing for AIDS globally, two-thirds for tuberculosis and three quarters for malaria.

- Global Health Council, http://www.globalhealth.org/.
  Created in 1972, the Global Health Council is the world's largest membership alliance dedicated to saving lives by improving health throughout the world. Its membership is comprised of health-care professionals and organizations that include NGOs, foundations, corporations, government agencies and academic institutions that work to ensure global health for all. It works to ensure that all who strive for improvement and equity in global health have the information and resources they need to succeed. The Council convenes the Malaria Roundtable, which is a community space where individuals and organizations dedicated to policies and programs that reduce the global burden of malaria can meet, exchange information and share resources.

- Friends of the Global Fight Against AIDS, Tuberculosis, and Malaria, http://www.theglobalfight.org/.
  Friends of the Global Fight Against AIDS, Tuberculosis and Malaria is an advocacy organization dedicated to sustaining and expanding U.S. support for the Global Fund's lifesaving work around the world. Created in 2004, Friends supports the Global Fund by raising awareness about its lifesaving work with policy leaders and decision makers in Washington, D.C., as well as the media and the advocacy community. The goal of these efforts is to achieve both sustained governmental funding and meaningful public policy on the Global Fund and the three diseases.

- Global Subsidies Initiative (GSI), http://www.globalsubsidies.org/en.
  In December 2005 the GSI was launched to put a spotlight on subsidies - transfers of public money to private interests - and how they undermine efforts to put the world economy on a path toward sustainable development. The GSI, in cooperation with a growing international network of research and media partners, seeks to lay bare just what good or harm public subsidies are doing; to encourage public debate and awareness of the options that are available; and to help provide policy-makers with the tools they need to secure sustainable outcomes for our societies and our planet.

- Innovative Vector Control Consortium, http://www.ivcc.com/.
  The IVCC is a major research consortium which will develop new and better ways to control the transmission of insect borne disease. Five

leading research institutions form the IVCC.[55] During the past three decades, there has been little progress in developing new insecticides for public health use in combating vectors (such as mosquitoes), which carry diseases such as malaria and dengue. The IVCC has been established to address problems such as the inefficient deployment of pesticides and the growth of pesticide-resistant insect strains by developing a portfolio of chemical and technological tools that will be immediately accessible to populations in the developing world.

- Institute of Medicine (IOM),
  The IOM's mission is to serve as adviser to the United States to improve health. A non-profit organization specifically created to provide science-based advice on matters of biomedical science, medicine, and health as well as an honorific membership organization, the IOM was chartered in 1970 as a component of the National Academy of Sciences. The Institute provides a vital service by working outside the framework of government to ensure scientifically informed analysis and independent guidance. The Institute provides unbiased, evidence-based, and authoritative information and advice concerning health and science policy to policymakers, professionals, leaders in every sector of society, and the public at large.

- Malaria Consortium, http://www.malariaconsortium.org/index.php.
  The Malaria Consortium is an organization dedicated to improving delivery of prevention and treatment to combat malaria and other communicable diseases in Africa and Asia. It works with communities, health systems, government and non-government agencies, academic institutions and local and international organizations, to ensure good evidence supports delivery of effective services. Started as a research center in 1992 working as part of the London School of Hygiene and Tropical Medicine, the Malaria Consortium became an independent NGO in 2003.

- Malaria Foundation International (MFI), http://www.malaria
  The MFI is a non-profit organization, dedicated to the fight against malaria since 1992. The MFI works in partnership with many individuals and groups who have since joined this cause. The MFI's goals are to support awareness, education, training, research, and leadership programs for the immediate and long term development and application of tools to combat malaria.

- Malaria-Measles Initiative, http://www.measlesinitiative.org/.

The Measles Initiative is a partnership committed to reducing measles deaths globally. Launched in 2001, the Initiative — led by the American Red Cross, the United Nations Foundation, CDC, UNICEF and WHO — provides technical and financial support to governments and communities on vaccination campaigns and disease surveillance worldwide. Measles vaccination campaigns usually include additional health services: for example, between 2001 and 2007, the Measles Initiative and its partners supported the distribution of more than 31 million insecticide-treated bed nets for malaria prevention.

- Malaria No More, http://www.malarianomore.org/.

Founded in 2006, Malaria No More is determined to end malaria deaths. A non-profit, nongovernmental organization, Malaria No More makes high-yield investments of time and capital to speed progress, unlock resources, mobilize new assets, and spur the world toward reaching this goal. The Malaria No More Policy Center works to raise awareness and galvanize support to address the global fight against malaria. Headquartered in Washington, D.C., the Center works with the global health community to engage policy leaders in the United States and in other donor nations to advance efforts to defeat malaria worldwide.

- Malaria R&D Alliance, http://www.malariaalliance.org/.

In March 2004, leaders and representatives of 15 organizations conducting malaria research and product development formed the Malaria R&D to raise awareness about the important role of malaria R&D in the malaria continuum and to develop a shared responsibility and increase resources for malaria R&D.

- Medicines for Malaria Venture (MMV), http://www.mmv.org/.

Medicines for Malaria Venture (MMV) is a non-profit organization created [in 1999] to discover, develop and deliver effective and affordable antimalarial drugs through public- private partnerships.

- Medicins Sans Frontieres (MSF), http://www.msf.org/.

MSF has been setting up emergency medical aid missions around the world since 1971. MSF is an international humanitarian aid organization that provides emergency medical assistance to populations in danger in more than 70 countries. In countries where health structures are insufficient or even non-existent, MSF collaborates with authorities such as the Ministry of Health to provide assistance. MSF works in rehabilitation of hospitals and dispensaries, vaccination programs, and water and sanitation projects. MSF also works in remote health care centers, slum areas and provides training of local personnel. All this is done with the objective of rebuilding health structures to acceptable levels. In carrying out humanitarian assistance, MSF seeks also to raise awareness of crisis situations.

- MIMCom (a project of the Multilateral Initiative on Malaria (MIM) and the U.S. National Library of Medicine (NLM)), *http://www. nlm. nih.gov/mimcom/mimcomhomepage.html.*

  MIMcom was conceived by African malaria researchers in 1997. The mandate for Internet access to medical literature came from African scientists: "Access to e-mail and the Internet will promote rapid communication between investigators working at different sites as well as access to online literature and data available to scientists outside Africa." Having established or enhanced connectivity at 21 research sites in 12 countries, NLM's current focus is on products and databases to aid the efforts of malaria research.

- Multilateral Initiative on Malaria (MIM), *http:// www. mimalaria. org/index.asp.*

  The Multilateral Initiative on Malaria (MIM) was established in 1997 with a mission to strengthen and sustain, through collaborative research and training, the capacity of malaria- endemic countries in Africa to carry out research that is required to develop and improve tools for malaria control and to strengthen the research-control interphase."

  Program for Appropriate Technology in Health (PATH) Malaria Vaccine Initiative (MVI), http://www.malariavaccine.org/.

  MVI was established in 1999 through a grant from the Bill & Melinda Gates Foundation . . . to accelerate the development of malaria vaccines and ensure their availability and accessibility in the developing world.

- Roll Back Malaria Partnership (RBM), http://www.rbm.who.int/.

  To provide a coordinated global approach to fighting malaria, the Roll Back Malaria (RBM) Partnership was launched in 1998 by the World Health Organization (WHO), the United Nations Children's Fund (UNICEF), the United Nations Development Programme (UNDP) and the World Bank. The RBM Partnership is now made up of a wide range of partners — including malaria-endemic countries, their bilateral and multilateral development partners, the private sector, non-governmental and community-based organizations, foundations, and research and academic institutions — who bring a formidable assembly of expertise, infrastructure and funds into the fight against the disease.

- Rotarians Eliminating Malaria – A Rotarian Action Group, http://www.remarag.org/.

  ReMaRAG, which was recognized by the Rotary International Board in 2005, functions as an umbrella association, building a network to keep tabs on Rotary projects in all corners of the world. The group has contacts in countries with malaria projects, and it acts as a resource to prevent duplication of efforts, promote best practices, and connect interested parties.

- UNICEF, http://www.unicef.org/health/index_malaria

  In recognition of its role as one of the biggest killers of children in Africa, malaria prevention and control interventions form an integral component of a minimum package of UNICEF's high impact maternal and child survival interventions. Integrated programming of this kind utilizes existing systems with relatively high utilization by target groups.

- UNITAID, http://www.unitaid.eu/index.php/en/.

  In 2006, UNITAID was created as an international drug purchase facility to be financed with sustainable, predictable resources in order to facilitate access to drugs for the world's poorest people as part of the fight against the major pandemic diseases. As an economically neutral tool, involved countries agreed a tax on international air tickets was the most suitable instrument for raising funds. This mechanism seeks to fill a critical gap in the global health financing landscape: the need for sustained strategic market intervention to drive price reduction and increases in supply.

- VOICES for a Malaria-Free Future, *http://www.malaria* freefuture. org/.

  VOICES for a Malaria-Free Future works to educate policymakers about effective programs and strategies for malaria control by highlighting successful anti-malaria efforts and evidence-based results. VOICES includes advocacy projects in four developing countries — Ghana, Kenya, Mali, and Mozambique — that promote progress made against malaria while also breaking down policy barriers that hamper effective prevention and control.

- World Bank Malaria Booster Program for Malaria Control in Africa, http://go.worldbank.org/H31FEKFWE0.

The Booster Program was launched in September 2005, translating the World Bank malaria global strategy into a results-focused effort to bring the disease under control on the African continent. The Booster Program has a ten-year horizon.

- WHO Global Collaboration for Development of Pesticides for Public Health (GCDPP), http://www.who.int/whopes/gcdpp/en/.

To strengthen WHO's Pesticides Evaluation Scheme (WHOPES) activities, to facilitate the search for alternative safe and more cost-effective pesticides and application methodologies, and to further promote the safe and proper use of pesticides and application equipment, WHOPES established the Global Collaboration for Development of Pesticides for Public Health (GCDPP). This collaboration provides a forum for exchange of information and ideas on issues related to the development and use of pesticides and pesticide application equipment within the context of WHO's global disease control strategies, and serves an advisory and resource-mobilizing role to WHOPES.

- WHO Global Malaria Programme (GMP), *http://www.* who.int/malaria

GMP is responsible for malaria policy and strategy formulation, operations support and capacity development, and coordination of WHO's global efforts to fight malaria. GMP establishes and promotes — based on evidence and expert consensus — WHO policies, normative standards and guidelines for malaria prevention and control, including monitoring and evaluation.

- WHO International Medical Products Anti-Counterfeiting Taskforce (IMPACT), http://www.who.int/impact/en/.

Responding to the growing public health crisis of counterfeit drugs, in February 2006, WHO launched IMPACT, which aims to build coordinated networks across and between countries in order to halt the production, trading and selling of fake medicines around the globe. IMPACT is a partnership comprised of all the major anti-counterfeiting players, including international organizations, NGOs, enforcement agencies, pharmaceutical manufacturers associations, and drug and regulatory authorities.

- WHO Tropical Disease Research (TDR), http://www.who.int/tdr/.

TDR, a Special Programme for Research and Training in Tropical Diseases, is an independent global programme of scientific collaboration that helps coordinate, support and influence global efforts to combat a portfolio of major diseases of the poor and disadvantaged. Established in 1975, TDR, is sponsored by UNICEF, the United Nations Development Programme (UNDP), the World Bank, and WHO. Its goal is to have the priority setting, research and development led and managed by scientific leaders in the countries where the diseases and problems occur. It believes this is a sustainable way of not only creating these tools, but making sure that they are distributed, used, and truly owned by the communities they can help.

End Notes

[1] Centers for Disease Control and Prevention (CDC), "Eradication of Malaria in the United States (1947-1951)," April 23, 2004; and World Health Organization (WHO), *World Malaria Report 2008*.

[2] For more information on U.S. government malaria research activities, which may receive funding through USAID, the Department of Health and Human Services (HHS), and the Department of Defense (DOD), see USAID, "Malaria," in *Health-Related Research and Development Activities at USAID: An Update on the Five-Year Strategy, 2006–2010*, Report to Congress, September 2008, pp. 37-40; *http://pdf.usaid.gov/* pdf_docs /PDACL916.pdf; CDC, "CDC Activities: Malaria Research," April 23, 2004, http://www.cdc.gov/malaria/cdcactivities/research.htm; HHS/National Institutes of Health (NIH), National Institute of Allergy and Infectious Diseases (NIAID) malaria research website, http://www3.niaid.nih.gov/topics/Malaria/research/; and DOD/Walter Reed Army Institute of Research (WRAIR) malaria website, *http://wrair-www.army.mil/* index. php? view=malaria.

[3] WHO, *The Global Burden of Disease: 2004 Update*, 2008; WHO, *World Malaria Report 2008*; and WHO/United Nations Children's Fund (UNICEF), *The Africa Malaria Report 2003*.

[4] There are four types of human malaria – *Plasmodium falciparum*, *P.vivax*, *P.malariae*, and *P.ovale*. *P.falciparum* and *P.vivax* are the most common. *P.falciparum* is the deadliest type of malaria infection.

[5] Based on WHO-recommended policies and strategies and the President's Malaria Initiative (PMI) approach.

[6] IPTp reduces the likelihood of malaria infection during pregnancy or, if the mother is infected, clears the malaria parasite from the placenta. Its use is recommended in areas with moderate to high levels of malaria transmission. WHO/Africa Regional Office, *Recommendations on the Use of Sulfadoxine-Pyrimethamine (SP) for Intermittent Preventive Treatment during Pregnancy (IPT) in Areas of Moderate to High Resistance to SP in the African Region*, October 2005.

[7] USAID, Report to Congress: Child Survival And Health Programs Fund Progress Report Fiscal Year 2007.

[8] WHO, *Global Malaria Control and Elimination: Report of a Technical Review*, January 17-18, 2008; and J.A. Najera, "Malaria and the Work of WHO," in *Bulletin of the World Health Organization*, Vol. 67, no. 3, 1989, pp. 229-243.

[9] U.N. General Assembly, Forty-Ninth Session, "Preventive Action and Intensification of the Struggle Against Malaria in Developing Countries, Particularly in Africa," A/RES/49/135, February 17, 1995. Organization of African Unity, *Declarations and Decisions Adopted by the Thirty-Third Assembly of Heads of State and Government*, June 2-4, 1997, AHG/Decl. 1

(XXXIII); and RBM/WHO, *The Abuja Declaration and the Plan of Action: An Extract from the African Summit on Roll Back Malaria, Abuja, 25 April 2000 (WHO/CDS/RBM/2000. 17)*, WHO/CDS/RBM/2003.46.

[10] United Nations, *United Nations Millennium Declaration*, A/RES/55/2, September 18, 2000. The goals and targets outlined in the document are often called the Millennium Development Goals (MDGs). The malaria goal is related to MDG 6, which focuses on combating HIV/AIDS, malaria, and other diseases, and is specified in Target 3. 58th World Health Assembly/WHO, *Resolutions and Decisions: WHA58.2, Malaria Control*, May 23, 2005. Resolution suggested by WHO, *Report by the Secretariat: A58/8, Malaria*, April 14, 2005.

[11] Additionally, in the Control Act, Congress recommends that the USAID Administrator consider the interaction of the HIV/AIDS, tuberculosis, and malaria epidemics, while in the Leadership Act, it states that a major objective of the U.S. foreign assistance program is to provide aid for the prevention, control, and cure of malaria.[11] These actions elevated malaria on the U.S. global health agenda, alongside HIV/AIDS and tuberculosis.

[12] House Committee on International Relations/ Subcommittee on Africa, Global Human Rights, and International Operations, "Malaria and Tuberculosis in Africa," H. Hrg. 108-141, September 14, 2004, 108th Congress, second session; Senate Committee on Foreign Relations/East Asia and Pacific Affairs Subcommittee, "Neglected Diseases in East Asia: Are Public Health Programs Working?," S. Hrg. 108-848, October 6, 2004, 108th Congress, second session; House Committee on International Relations/ Subcommittee on Africa, Global Human Rights, and International Operations, "Malaria and TB: Implementing Proven Treatment and Eradication Methods," H. Hrg. 109-65, April 26, 2005, 109th Congress, first session; Senate Committee on Homeland Security and Governmental Affairs/Federal Financial Management, Government Information, and International Security Subcommittee, "Examining USAID's Anti-Malaria Policies," S. Hrg. 109-139, May 12, 2005, 109th Congress, first session; and Elimination of Neglected Diseases Act of 2005 (S. 950, not enacted). S. 950 proposed establishing a U.S. global malaria coordinator, requiring a five-year U.S. global malaria strategy, and increasing spending on commodities while limiting spending on technical assistance.

[13] Opening statement of Senator Tom Coburn in S. Hrg. 109-13 9.

[14] PMI, "USAID Malaria Program Inputs FY2004," and "Malaria Program Inputs FY2005," http://fightingmalaria.gov/funding

[15] USAID, "Section II: Restructuring of USAID Malaria Programs," in *FY 2006 Report to Committees on Appropriations: USAID Malaria Programming, Report No. 1*, February 2006; and USAID/CDC Interagency Working Group, "President's Malaria Initiative Strategic Plan," July 25, 2005.

[16] George W. Bush Administration, "Fighting Malaria in Africa," press release, June 30, 2005. This goal reflects international goals for malaria control, such as the RBM goal of reducing the global malaria burden by 50% by 2010. RBM, *Consolidating Progress and Moving to Scale With Action in Countries*, 3rd Meeting of the Global Partnership Roll Back Malaria, February 2-3, 2000, WHO/CDS/RBM/2000. 13, Geneva, Switzerland, April 2000.

[17] See **Appendix C** for more information.

[18] USAID, "Section II: Restructuring of USAID Malaria Programs," in *FY 2006 Report to Committees on Appropriations: USAID Malaria Programming, Report No. 1*, February 2006.

[19] Comments by Admiral Tim Ziemer, U.S. Global Malaria Coordinator, congressional briefing, February 27, 2009.

[20] Senate Committee on Homeland Security and Governmental Affairs/Federal Financial Management, Government Information, and International Security Subcommittee, "Bilateral Malaria Assistance: Progress and Prognosis," S. Hrg. 109-614, January 19, 2006, 109th Congress, second session.

[21] For more information, see CRS Report RL34569, *PEPFAR Reauthorization: Key Policy Debates and Changes to U.S. International HIV/AIDS, Tuberculosis, and Malaria Programs and Funding*, by Kellie Moss.

[22] Comments made by then Senator Obama during the 2008 annual meeting of the Clinton Global Initiative, September 25, 2008. This goal is similar to one set in RBM, *The Global Malaria Action Plan: For A Malaria-Free World*, 2008.

[23] Office of Management and Budget (OMB), "Department of State and Other International Programs," *A New Era of Responsibility: Renewing America's Promise*, FY20 10 Budget.

[24] PMI, *Saving the Lives of Mothers and Children in Africa*, First Annual Report, March 2007; PMI, *Progress Through Partnerships: Saving Lives in Africa*, Second Annual Report, March 2008; PMI, "Fast Facts: The President's Malaria Initiative," April 2008; and CRS Correspondence with PMI staff, March 6, 2009.

[25] PMI implementing agencies report that they set this PMI target in order to achieve the overall goal of reducing the number of malaria-related deaths in the 15 PMI countries by 50% by 2010. PMI, Second Annual Report, March 2008.

[26] See **Appendix C** for more information.

[27] According to CDC, malaria may be diagnosed as uncomplicated or complicated (severe). Severe malaria occurs when *P. falciparum* infections are complicated by serious organ failures or abnormalities in the patient's blood or metabolism. See CDC, "Malaria: Disease," September 21, 2006.

[28] These efforts are sometimes part of an integrated approach to maternal and child health called Focused Antenatal Care (FANC), which is recommended by WHO. WHO states that FANC is a package of interventions usually provided over four antenatal care visits. Some of the services it includes are IPTp, immunizations, identification and management of infections such as tuberculosis and syphilis, counseling, prevention of mother-to-child HIV transmission [PMTCT], identification and management of obstetric complications such as pre-eclampsia, and birth preparedness. See WHO, *Department of Making Pregnancy Safer Annual Report 2007*.

[29] PMI, First Annual Report, March 2007.

[30] For more information on PEPFAR, see CRS Report RL34569 , PEPFAR Reauthorization: Key Policy Debates and Changes to U.S. International HIV/AIDS, Tuberculosis, and Malaria Programs and Funding, by Kellie Moss.

[31] The seven countries in which PEPFAR and PMI both operate are Ethiopia, Kenya, Mozambique, Rwanda, Tanzania, Uganda, and Zambia.

[32] For descriptions of and weblinks to the organizations listed above, as well as other key malaria organizations, see **Appendix D**. For more information on the Global Fund, see CRS Report RL33396, *The Global Fund to Fight AIDS, Tuberculosis, and Malaria: Progress Report and Issues for Congress*, by Tiaji Salaam-Blyther and CRS Report RL3 1712, The Global Fund to Fight AIDS, Tuberculosis, and Malaria: Background, by Tiaji Salaam-Blyther.

[33] PMI Malaria Communities Program website, http://fightingmalaria.gov/about/mcp/aboutmcp.html.

[34] Based on CRS Correspondence with Dr. Trent Ruebush, Senior Malaria Advisor, USAID Bureau for Global Health, November 7, 2008; USAID malaria overview website, http://www.usaid.gov/our_work/global_health/id/malaria/; USAID, "Section II: Restructuring of USAID Malaria Programs," in *FY 2006 Report to Committees on Appropriations: USAID Malaria Programming, Report No. 1*, February 2006; USAID, "USAID Provides Malaria Assistance to Zimbabwe," press release, February 11, 2009; and USAID, *Report to Congress: Child Survival and Health Programs Fund Progress Report Fiscal Year 2007*.

[35] Based on CRS Correspondence with CDC, March 6, 2009; CRS Correspondence with CDC, March 11, 2009; CRS Conversation with CDC staff, November 5, 2008; CDC, international malaria activities webpages, http://www.cdc.gov/malaria/cdcactivities/index.htm.

[36] CDC, "CDC Role in the President's Malaria Initiative," provided to CRS by CDC, September 23, 2008.

[37] For more information on CDC's global malaria program, see CRS Report R40239, *Centers for Disease Control and Prevention Global Health Programs: FY2004-FY2009*, by Tiaji Salaam-Blyther.

[38] Since the creation of PMI, USAID's funding for malaria programs has shifted from smaller amounts of funding for many countries to greater amounts for fewer countries and selected regional and central programs. See **Appendix C** for data on USAID funding by program, including funding for PMI and other USAID malaria programs.

[39] Founded in 2002, the Global Fund to Fight AIDS, Tuberculosis, and Malaria (Global Fund) is the largest global funder of malaria programs worldwide. It is an international financing mechanism, not an implementing agency, that is supported by donor contributions. The Global Fund distributes contributed funds periodically through "rounds" in its grants process, which awards grants for projects that fight HIV/AIDS, tuberculosis, malaria, or a combination of these diseases; or that engage in health systems strengthening. For more information on Global Fund spending by disease, see Global Fund website on "Distribution of Funding After 7 Rounds By Disease," *http://www.theglobalfund.org/* en/ distributionfunding/.

[40] Perspectives included in this section are based on CRS interviews and discussions with malaria and global health experts and staff from NGOs; think tanks; universities; international organizations; a private sector medical research institution; and U.S. government departments, agencies, and offices.

[41] For more information, see CRS Report RS22913, *Global Health: Appropriations to USAID Programs from FY2001 through FY2008*, by Tiaji Salaam-Blyther.

[42] S. Hrg. 109-139.

[43] Kenneth J. Arrow, Claire Panosian, and Hellen Gelband, eds., Institute of Medicine Committee on the Economics of Antimalarial Drugs, *Saving Lives, Buying Time: Economics of Malaria Drugs in an Age of Resistance*, July 20, 2004.

[44] One proposed mechanism for such a subsidy that the United States might support, some argue, is the Affordable Medicines Facility—malaria (AMFm), which the Global Fund may host within its structure. However, in the Lantos- Hyde Act (P.L. 110-293), Congress states that the Global Fund should not support activities involving AMFm or similar entities until the U.S. Global Malaria Coordinator evaluates pilot programs and finds "compelling evidence of success." Global Fund, "Report of the Affordable Medicines Facility—Malaria Ad Hoc Committee," GF/B18/7 Decision, 18th Board Meeting, November 7-8, 2008.

[45] WHO, *Global Malaria Control and Elimination: Report of a Meeting on Containment of Artemisinin Tolerance,* January 19, 2008; and WHO, *Technical Expert Group Meeting on Intermittent Preventive Treatment in Pregnancy (IPTp)*, July 11-13, 2007.

[46] MSF, *Full Prescription: Better Malaria Treatment for More People, MSF's Experience*, September 2008.

[47] WHO, "Malaria," Fact Sheet No. 94, May 2007; and Roger Bate, "New Insecticides Are Crucial in Battle Against Malaria," AEI.org, February 19, 2009.

[48] For more information, see Roger Bate, *Making a Killing: The Deadly Implications of the Counterfeit Drug Trade*, AEI Press, Washington, May 2008.

[49] For more information on DDT use in malaria control, see Richard Tren and Roger Bate, *Malaria and the DDT Story*, Institute of Economic Affairs, 2001. For more information on the EU insecticide debate, see "Regulating Pesticides: A Balance of Risk," *The Economist*, July 3, 2008; and Jasson Urbach, "New EU Pesticide Legislation Threatens African Malaria Control Initiatives," HealthPolicyUnit.com, January 19, 2009. For more information on insecticides and their role in malaria control, see Africa Fighting Malaria, *Bias & Neglect: Public Health Insecticides & Disease Control*, December 2008.

[50] Some opponents of disease-specific initiatives argue that recent efforts like PMI and PEPFAR have negatively impacted USAID's ability to carry out other health sector efforts, such as

maternal and child health programs. In FY2004, for example, USAID malaria funding was less than 5% of its global health budget, excluding U.S. contributions to the Global Fund. By FY2008, malaria funding was almost 17% of USAID's global health budget, excluding U.S. contributions to the Global Fund.

[51] One study that appeared in *The Lancet* reported that "many health ministries have become donor dependent." It cited the cases of Tanzania, Kenya, and Uganda, whose health ministers reported that 40% to 60% of their ministries' budgets come from donors. See D. Sridhar and R. Batniji, "Misfinancing Global Health: A Case for Transparency in Disbursements and Decision Making," *The Lancet*, Volume 372, Issue 9644, pp. 1185–1191.

[52] Global Fund, *Board of the Global Fund*,
http://www.theglobalfund.org/en/board/?lang=en.

[53] Calculated by CRS by averaging the percentage of funding spent on commodities in each of the 15 PMI countries for each fiscal year, based on PMI Malaria Operational Plans, http://fightingmalaria.gov/countries/mops/index.html.

[54] These are "five public sector institutions – the Oswaldo Cruz Foundation from Brazil, the Indian Council for Medical Research, the Kenya Medical Research Institute, the Ministry of Health of Malaysia and France's Pasteur Institute; one humanitarian organisation, Médecins sans Frontières (MSF); and one international research organisation, the UNDP/World Bank/WHO's Special Programme for Research and Training in Tropical Diseases (TDR), which acts as a permanent observer to the initiative." See DNDi, "About DNDi," http://www.dndi.org/cms/public_html/insidearticleListing.asp?CategoryId=87&ArticleId=288&TemplateId=1.

[55] These are the Liverpool School of Tropical Medicine; the London School of Hygiene and Tropical Medicine; University of California at Davis, California; Colorado State University; and the Medical Research Council, South Africa.

In: Understanding Malaria and Lyme Disease   ISBN: 978-1-61761-435-4
Editors: Kristen C. Walsch   © 2010 Nova Science Publishers, Inc.

Chapter 3

LYME DISEASE: THE FACTS AND THE CHALLENGE

U.S. Department of Health and Human Services

INTRODUCTION

In the early 1970s, a mysterious clustering of arthritis cases occurred among children in Lyme, Connecticut, and surrounding towns. Puzzled medical experts eventually labeled the illness as a new disease, which they called Lyme disease. By the mid-1970s, scientists were busy describing signs and symptoms of Lyme disease to help doctors diagnose patients. Scientists eventually learned that antibiotics were an effective treatment, and that the bite of the deer tick was the key to the spread of disease.

None of these findings, however, happened overnight. In fact, it wasn't until 1981—through a bit of puzzle solving and keen recollection—that the cause of Lyme disease was identified and the connection between the deer tick and the disease was discovered.

Lyme disease is still mistaken for other illnesses, and it continues to pose many other challenges, including the following:

It can be difficult to diagnose.
It can be hard to treat in its later phases.

A number of different ticks can transmit diseases with symptoms like
   Lyme disease.
Deer ticks can pass on diseases other than Lyme disease.

This booklet presents the most recently available information on the
diagnosis, treatment, and prevention of Lyme disease.

Note: Words in bold are defined in the glossary near the end of this
booklet.

HOW LYME DISEASE BECAME KNOWN

Lyme disease was first recognized in 1975 after researchers tried to find
out why unusually large numbers of children were being diagnosed with
juvenile rheumatoid arthritis in Lyme, Connecticut, and two neighboring
towns. After considering several possible causes, such as contact with germs
(**microbes**) in water or air, researchers focused their attention on deer ticks.
They realized that most of the affected children lived and played near wooded
areas.

Researchers knew that the children's first symptoms typically started
during summer—the height of tick season. Several of the children reported
having a skin rash just before developing their arthritis. Many of them recalled
being bitten by a tick where the rash appeared.

Before Lyme Disease Became Known

Around the same time, about 2,500 miles away from Lyme, Willy
Burgdorfer, Ph.D., was conducting research at Rocky Mountain Laboratories
(RML) in Hamilton, Montana, part of the National Institute of Allergy and
Infectious Diseases (NIAID). Dr. Burgdorfer was studying Rocky Mountain
spotted fever, which is also caused by the bite of a tick.

In the summer of 1977, Allen C. Steere, M.D., was investigating the Lyme
disease cases for the Yale University School of Medicine in Hartford,
Connecticut. During conversations with Dr. Burgdorfer, Dr. Steere mentioned
the deer tick as the likely carrier for Lyme disease.

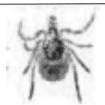

Ticks that most often transmit *B. burgdorferi* in the United States:
Isodes scapularis—most common in the Northeast and Midwest. Also found in the South and Southeast.
Ixodes pacificus—found on the West Coast.
These two ticks look quite similar.

Researchers in Europe had written about a skin rash similar to that of Lyme disease in medical literature dating back to the turn of the 20th century. Dr. Burgdorfer wondered if the European rash, called erythema migrans, and Lyme disease might have the same cause.

As Dr. Burgdorfer and his RML colleague Alan Barbour, M.D., continued to study spiral-shaped bacteria, or spirochetes, from infected deer ticks, they eventually achieved success. In late November 1981, the scientists found the cause of both Lyme disease and the European skin rash. The spirochete was later named *Borrelia burgdorferi* in honor of Dr. Burgdorfer for his role in discovering it.

Although Lyme disease may have spread from Europe to the United States in the early 1900s, health experts only recently recognized it as a distinct illness.

Deer Ticks

Small rodents and deer play an important role in a deer tick's life cycle. Today, scientists who study Lyme disease are learning much more about that role.

Both nymphs (immature ticks) and adult ticks can transmit Lyme disease-causing bacteria. The recent increase of the deer population in the Northeast, and of housing developments in rural areas where deer ticks are commonly found, probably have contributed to the spread of the disease.

The numbers of cases of Lyme disease and of geographic areas in which it is found have increased. Healthcare providers have seen cases of Lyme disease in nearly all states in the United States. However, most reported cases are concentrated in the coastal Northeast, the mid-Atlantic states, Wisconsin, Minnesota, and northern California. Lyme disease is also found in large areas of Asia and Europe.

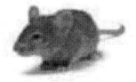

- Deer ticks lay eggs that turn into larvae that feed on mice and other small mammals.
- The larvae then develop into immature ticks called nymphs.
- The nymphs then feed on small mammals and humans.
- Adult deer ticks usually feed on deer during the adult part of their life cycles.

SYMPTOMS OF LYME DISEASE

Erythema Migrans

Erythema migrans (EM) is usually the first symptom of Lyme disease.

The telltale rash starts as a small red spot at the site of the tick bite.
The spot gets larger over a period of days or weeks and forms a red rash shaped like a circle or an oval.

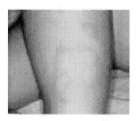

Sometimes the rash looks like a bull's eye, appearing as a red ring surrounding a clear area with a red center. The rash, which can range in size from that of a small coin to the width of your back, appears within a few weeks of a tick bite and usually at the place of the bite. As infection spreads, rashes can appear at different places on the body.

Other symptoms that often appear with EM can include:

- Fever
- Headache
- Stiff neck
- Body aches
- Tiredness

Although these symptoms may be like those of common viral infections such as the flu, Lyme disease symptoms tend to continue longer or may come and go.

Arthritis

After several months of infection with Lyme bacteria, slightly more than half of people not treated with antibiotics develop recurrent attacks of painful and swollen joints. These attacks last a few days to a few months. The arthritis can move from one joint to another. The knee is most commonly affected.

About 10 to 20 percent of people who have not taken antibiotics will go on to develop chronic (long-lasting) arthritis.

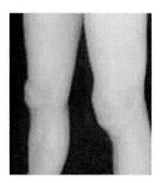

Neurological Symptoms

Lyme disease can also affect your nervous system, causing symptoms such as the following:

- Stiff neck and severe headache (meningitis)
- Temporary paralysis of your facial muscles (Bell's palsy)
- Numbness, pain, or weakness in your limbs
- Poor muscle movement

Lyme disease can also cause more subtle changes such as

- Memory loss
- Difficulty with concentration
- Change in mood or sleep habits

Neurological problems usually develop several weeks, months, or even years following untreated infection. These symptoms often last for weeks or months and may return.

Less commonly, people who have not taken antibiotics may develop heart or other problems weeks, months, or even years after they were infected with Lyme bacteria.

Heart Problems

Fewer than 1 out of 10 people with Lyme disease develop heart problems, such as irregular heartbeat, which can start with dizziness or shortness of breath. These symptoms rarely last more than a few days or weeks. Such heart problems generally show up several weeks after a person is infected with Lyme bacteria.

Other Symptoms

Less commonly, Lyme disease can cause eye
inflammation, hepatitis (liver disease), and severe fatigue. None of these problems, however, is likely to appear without other Lyme disease symptoms being present.

HOW LYME DISEASE IS DIAGNOSED

Your healthcare provider may have difficulty diagnosing Lyme disease because many of its symptoms are similar to those of other illnesses. In addition, the only symptom that is unique to Lyme disease is the rash. That rash is absent in at least one-fourth of the people who become infected.

The results of recent research studies show that an infected tick must be attached to the skin for at least 2 days to transmit Lyme bacteria. Although a tick bite is an important clue for diagnosis, many people cannot recall having been bitten recently by a tick. This is not surprising because the deer tick is tiny, and a tick bite is usually painless.

If you have Lyme disease symptoms, but do not develop the distinctive rash, your healthcare provider will rely on a detailed medical history and a careful physical exam for clues to diagnose it. You will also be given laboratory tests to help diagnose the disease.

Medical History

If you don't have the EM rash, your healthcare provider will diagnose Lyme disease based on

- Whether your symptoms first appeared during the summer months when tick bites are most likely to occur
- Whether you were outdoors in an area where Lyme disease is common
- Whether you have been bitten by a tick
- Whether you have other symptoms of Lyme disease

In addition, your healthcare provider will rule out other diseases that might be causing your symptoms.

Lab Tests

It is difficult for healthcare providers to find the bacterium that causes Lyme disease in lab tests of body **tissues** or fluids. Therefore, most look for evidence of **antibodies** against *B. burgdorferi* in the blood to confirm that the bacterium is causing the symptoms.

Healthcare providers cannot always find out whether Lyme disease bacteria absolutely are causing symptoms. In the first few weeks following infection, antibody tests are not reliable because your **immune system** has not produced enough antibodies to be found. Antibiotics given early during infection may also prevent antibodies from reaching levels that a test can find, even though Lyme disease bacteria are causing your symptoms.

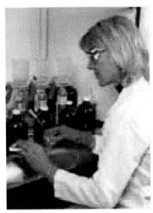

The antibody test most often used is called an ELISA (*e*nzyme-*l*inked *i*mmuno*s*orbent *a*ssay) test. The Food and Drug Administration (FDA) has approved two antibody tests:

- Prevue B, a rapid test, can give results within an hour.
- The C6 Lyme Peptide ELISA is very sensitive and specific.

If your ELISA is positive, your healthcare provider should confirm it with a second, more specific test called a Western blot.

If you have nervous system symptoms, you may also get a spinal tap. Using this test, your healthcare provider can find any inflammation in your brain and spinal cord and can look for antibodies or genetic material of *B. burgdorferi* in your spinal fluid.

FDA has not approved tests for Lyme disease that use urine or some other body fluids to diagnose infection caused by Lyme bacteria.

New Tests being Developed

Healthcare providers need tests to tell apart people who have recovered from previous Lyme infection and those who continue to suffer from active infection.

To improve the accuracy of diagnosing Lyme disease, National Institutes of Health (NIH)-supported researchers are re-evaluating current tests. They are also developing a number of new tests that promise to be more reliable than those currently available.

NIH-supported scientists are developing tests that use the highly sensitive genetic engineering technique known as PCR (polymerase chain reaction) as well as **microarray** and **high-throughput genomic sequencing technology** to detect extremely small quantities of the genetic material of the Lyme disease bacterium or its products in body tissues and fluids.

A bacterial protein, outer surface protein (Osp) C, is proving useful for detecting specific antibodies early in people with Lyme disease. Because researchers have determined the **genome** of *B. burgdorferi*, there are now new avenues for improving their understanding of the disease and its diagnosis.

HOW LYME DISEASE IS TREATED

Using antibiotics appropriately, your healthcare provider can effectively treat your Lyme disease. In general, the sooner you begin treatment after you have been infected, the quicker and more complete your recovery.

Antibiotics such as doxycycline, cefuroxime axetil, or amoxicillin, taken orally for a few weeks, can speed the healing of the EM rash and usually prevent symptoms such as arthritis or neurological problems.

Doctors usually treat Lyme disease in children younger than 9 years, or in pregnant or breast-feeding women, with amoxicillin, cefuroxime axetil, or penicillin. They do not use doxycycline in these groups because the antibiotic can stain the permanent teeth developing in young children or unborn babies.

Arthritis

If you have Lyme arthritis, your healthcare provider may treat you with oral antibiotics. If your arthritis is severe, you may be given ceftriaxone or penicillin intravenously (through a vein). To ease any discomfort and to help with healing, your healthcare provider might also do one of the following:

- Give you anti-inflammatory drugs
- Draw fluid from your affected joints
- Perform surgery to remove the inflamed lining of those joints

In most people, Lyme arthritis goes away within a few weeks or months following antibiotic treatment. In some, however, it can take years to disappear completely. Some people with Lyme disease who are untreated for several years may be cured of their arthritis with the proper antibiotic treatment.

The disease, however, does not always go away with treatment. If it has lasted long enough, it may permanently damage the structure of your joints.

Neurological Problems

If you have neurological symptoms, your healthcare provider will probably treat you with the antibiotic ceftriaxone given intravenously once a day for a month or less. Most people recover completely.

Heart Problems

Healthcare providers prefer to treat people with Lyme disease who have heart symptoms with antibiotics such as ceftriaxone or penicillin given intravenously for about 2 weeks. People with Lyme disease rarely have long-term heart damage.

Problems after Treatment

Following treatment for Lyme disease, you might still have muscle aches, and neurological problems such as tiredness and trouble with memory and concentration.

NIH-sponsored researchers are doing research to find out the cause of these symptoms and the best ways to treat them. Research studies suggest that people who suffer from post-Lyme disease symptoms may be **genetically predisposed** to develop an **autoimmune** response that contributes to their symptoms. Researchers are now examining the significance of this finding in greater detail.

Researchers also are trying to find out the best length of time to give antibiotics for the various symptoms of Lyme disease.

Unfortunately, having a bout with Lyme disease once is no guarantee that you will not get the illness again. It can strike more than once if you are reinfected with Lyme disease bacteria.

How Lyme Disease Is Prevented

Avoid Ticks

At present, the best way you can avoid Lyme disease is to avoid deer ticks. Although generally only about 1 percent of all deer ticks are infected with Lyme disease bacteria, in some areas more than half of the ticks have the microbes.

More people with Lyme disease become infected during the summer, when immature ticks are found most often. In warm climates, deer ticks thrive and bite during the winter months as well.

- Spray insect repellant with 20 to 30 percent DEET (a chemical) on exposed skin and clothing to prevent tick bites.
- Spray clothing with permethrin, a repellant commonly found in lawn and garden stores. Permethrin kills ticks on contact. You should not apply permethrin directly to your skin.
- Wear long pants, long sleeves, and long socks to keep ticks off your skin. Light-colored clothing will help you spot ticks more easily. Tucking pant legs into socks or boots and tucking shirts into pants help keep ticks on the outside of your clothing. If you'll be outside for a long time, tape the area where your pants and socks meet to prevent ticks from crawling under your clothes.

Source: Centers for Disease Control and Prevention, National Center for Zoonotic, Vector-Borne, and Enteric Diseases

Deer ticks are most often found in wooded areas and nearby shady grasslands, and are especially common where the two areas merge. Because adult ticks feed on deer, areas where deer are seen frequently are likely to have large numbers of deer ticks.

If you are pregnant, be especially careful to avoid ticks in Lyme disease areas because you can pass on the infection to your unborn child.

Repellants, although highly effective, can cause some serious side effects, particularly when you put high concentrations on your skin over and over again. Infants and children especially may suffer from bad reactions to insect repellants containing DEET. If you repeatedly apply such repellants with concentrations of DEET higher than 15 percent, you should wash your skin, and any clothing, with soap and water.

Check for Ticks

The immature deer ticks most likely to cause Lyme disease are only about the size of a poppy seed, so they are easily mistaken for a freckle or a speck of dirt. Once indoors

- Check for ticks, particularly in the hairy regions of your body.
- Wash all clothing.
- Check pets for ticks before letting them inside.

Pets can carry ticks into the house. These ticks could fall off without biting the animal and then attach to and bite people. In addition, pets can develop symptoms of Lyme disease.

Studies by NIH-supported researchers suggest that a tick must be attached to the body for at least 48 hours to transmit Lyme disease bacteria. Promptly removing the tick could keep you from getting infected.

The risk of developing Lyme disease from a tick bite is small, even in heavily infested areas. Most healthcare providers prefer not to use antibiotics to treat people bitten by ticks unless they develop symptoms of Lyme disease.

Remove a tick from your skin as soon as you notice it. Use fine-tipped tweezers to firmly grasp the tick very close to your skin. With a steady motion, pull the tick's body away from your skin. Then clean your skin with soap and warm water. Throw the dead tick away with your household trash.

Avoid crushing the tick's body. Do not be alarmed if the tick's mouthparts remain in the skin. Once the mouthparts are removed from the rest of the tick, it can no longer transmit Lyme disease bacteria. If you accidentally crush the tick, clean your skin with soap and warm water or alcohol.

Don't use petroleum jelly, a hot match, nail polish, or other products to remove a tick.

Source: Centers for Disease Control and Prevention, National Center for Zoonotic, Vector-Borne, and Enteric Diseases

Get Rid of Ticks

Deer provide a safe haven for ticks that transmit *B. burgdorferi* and other disease-causing microbes. You can reduce the number of ticks, which can spread diseases in your area, by clearing trees and removing yard litter and excess brush that attract deer and rodents.

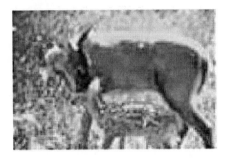

In the meantime, researchers are trying to develop an effective strategy for ridding areas of deer ticks. Studies show that spraying pesticides in wooded areas in the spring and fall can substantially reduce for more than a year the number of adult deer ticks living there. Spraying on a large scale, however, may not be economically feasible and may prompt environmental or health concerns.

Researchers also are testing pesticide-treated deer and rodent feeders as a possibly safer alternative for the environment. Tests done by the Centers for Disease Control and Prevention suggest that at least one commercial product reduced the number of ticks in the landscape by 80 percent during the first year of use and 97 percent by the second year.

Successful control of deer ticks will probably depend on a combination of tactics. Before strategies for wide-scale tick control can be put into practice, there needs to be more research.

RESEARCH: THE KEY TO PROGRESS

NIH conducts and supports biomedical research aimed at meeting the challenges of Lyme disease. Part of this research continues at NIAID' s Rocky Mountain Laboratories, where Dr. Burgdorfer performed his original work.

Scientists are gaining a better understanding of the human **immune response** that leads to Lyme disease. For example, they are uncovering what causes treatment- resistant Lyme arthritis. Improved understanding of the human immune response may lead to better diagnostic and **prognostic** tools. For example, the *B. burgdorferi* immune complex assay, a test being developed, shows active Lyme disease infection earlier than current antibody tests.

Because Lyme disease is difficult to diagnose and may not respond to treatment, researchers are trying to create a vaccine that will protect people from getting infected. Vaccines work in part by prompting the body to make antibodies. These custom-shaped **molecules** lock onto specific proteins made by a virus or bacterium. Often, those proteins lodge in the microbe's outer coat. Once antibodies attach to an invading microbe, other immune system defenses are called upon to destroy it.

Although Lyme disease poses many challenges, they are challenges the medical research community is well equipped to meet. New information on Lyme disease is accumulating at a rapid pace, thanks to the scientific research being conducted around the world.

GLOSSARY

antibody–a molecule tailor-made by the immune system to lock onto and destroy specific germs

autoimmune–when the immune system mistakenly attacks the body's own organs and tissues

gene–a unit of genetic material that carries the directions a cell uses to perform a specific function

genetic predisposition–when a person has alterations in the genes of his or her cells which increase the risk of developing a disease

genome–the sum of all the genetic materials in any organism

high-throughput genomic sequencing–a biomedical process used to rapidly determine the order of nucleotides (parts of DNA and RNA) in multiple DNA samples. (DNA and RNA are molecules that contain genetic information.)

immune response–the reaction of the immune system to foreign substances such as bacteria

immune system–a complex network of specialized cells, tissues, and organs that defends the body against attacks by "foreign" invaders

inflammation–a process of the immune system, with signs like redness and swelling, often seen at the site of an injury such as a tick bite

microarray–a tool used by scientists to analyze genomic information to understand how large numbers of genes are expressed or how they undergo changes to specific genetic sequences

microbe–the smallest forms of life, including bacteria, viruses, fungi, and parasites

molecule–a building block of a cell, such as proteins, fats, and carbohydrates

prognostic–having the ability to predict or forecast the outcome (prognosis) of a disease

tissue–a group of similar cells joined to perform the same function

CHAPTER SOURCES

The following chapters have been previously published:

Chapter 1 – This is an edited, reformatted U.S. Department of Health and Human Services National Institutes of Health publication No. 07-7139, dated February, 2007

Chapter 2 – This is an edited, reformatted and augmented version of Congressional Research Service publication, Report R40494, dated April 6, 2009.

Chapter 3 – This is an edited, reformatted U.S. Department of Health and Human Services National Institutes of Health publication No. 08-7045, dated July, 2008.

INDEX